Psychiatry: A Very Short Introduction

APPLIED MATHEMATICS
Alain Goriely
THE APOCRYPHAL GOSPELS
Paul Foster
ARCHAEOLOGY Paul Bahn
ARCHITECTURE Andrew Ballantyne
ARISTOCRACY William Doyle
ARISTOTLE Jonathan Barnes
ART HISTORY Dana Arnold
ART THEORY Cynthia Freeland
ARTIFICIAL INTELLIGENCE
Margaret A. Boden
ASIAN AMERICAN HISTORY
Madeline Y. Hsu
ASTROBIOLOGY David C. Catling
ASTROPHYSICS James Binney
ATHEISM Julian Baggini
THE ATMOSPHERE Paul I. Palmer
AUGUSTINE Henry Chadwick
AUSTRALIA Kenneth Morgan
AUTISM Uta Frith
AUTOBIOGRAPHY Laura Marcus
THE AVANT GARDE David Cottington
THE AZTECS Davíd Carrasco
BABYLONIA Trevor Bryce
BACTERIA Sebastian G. B. Amyes
BANKING John Goddard and
John O. S. Wilson
BARTHES Jonathan Culler
THE BEATS David Sterritt
BEAUTY Roger Scruton
BEHAVIOURAL ECONOMICS
Michelle Baddeley
BESTSELLERS John Sutherland
THE BIBLE John Riches
BIBLICAL ARCHAEOLOGY Eric H. Cline
BIG DATA Dawn E. Holmes
BIOGRAPHY Hermione Lee
BLACK HOLES Katherine Blundell
BLOOD Chris Cooper
THE BLUES Elijah Wald
THE BODY Chris Shilling
THE BOOK OF COMMON
PRAYER Brian Cummings
THE BOOK OF MORMON
Terryl Givens
BORDERS Alexander C. Diener and
Joshua Hagen
THE BRAIN Michael O'Shea
BRANDING Robert Jones
THE BRICS Andrew F. Cooper
THE BRITISH CONSTITUTION
Martin Loughlin
THE BRITISH EMPIRE Ashley Jackson
BRITISH POLITICS Anthony Wright
BUDDHA Michael Carrithers
BUDDHISM Damien Keown
BUDDHIST ETHICS Damien Keown
BYZANTIUM Peter Sarris
CALVINISM Jon Balserak
CANCER Nicholas James
CAPITALISM James Fulcher
CATHOLICISM Gerald O'Collins
CAUSATION Stephen Mumford and
Rani Lill Anjum
THE CELL Terence Allen and
Graham Cowling
THE CELTS Barry Cunliffe
CHAOS Leonard Smith
CHEMISTRY Peter Atkins
CHILD PSYCHOLOGY Usha Goswami
CHILDREN'S LITERATURE
Kimberley Reynolds
CHINESE LITERATURE Sabina Knight
CHOICE THEORY Michael Allingham
CHRISTIAN ART Beth Williamson
CHRISTIAN ETHICS D. Stephen Long
CHRISTIANITY Linda Woodhead
CIRCADIAN RHYTHMS Russell Foster
and Leon Kreitzman
CITIZENSHIP Richard Bellamy
CIVIL ENGINEERING
David Muir Wood
CLASSICAL LITERATURE William Allan
CLASSICAL MYTHOLOGY
Helen Morales
CLASSICS Mary Beard and
John Henderson
CLAUSEWITZ Michael Howard
CLIMATE Mark Maslin
CLIMATE CHANGE Mark Maslin
CLINICAL PSYCHOLOGY
Susan Llewelyn and
Katie Aafjes-van Doorn
COGNITIVE NEUROSCIENCE
Richard Passingham
THE COLD WAR Robert McMahon
COLONIAL AMERICA Alan Taylor
COLONIAL LATIN AMERICAN
LITERATURE Rolena Adorno

COMBINATORICS Robin Wilson
COMEDY Matthew Bevis
COMMUNISM Leslie Holmes
COMPARATIVE LITERATURE Ben Hutchinson
COMPLEXITY John H. Holland
THE COMPUTER Darrel Ince
COMPUTER SCIENCE Subrata Dasgupta
CONFUCIANISM Daniel K. Gardner
THE CONQUISTADORS Matthew Restall and Felipe Fernández-Armesto
CONSCIENCE Paul Strohm
CONSCIOUSNESS Susan Blackmore
CONTEMPORARY ART Julian Stallabrass
CONTEMPORARY FICTION Robert Eaglestone
CONTINENTAL PHILOSOPHY Simon Critchley
COPERNICUS Owen Gingerich
CORAL REEFS Charles Sheppard
CORPORATE SOCIAL RESPONSIBILITY Jeremy Moon
CORRUPTION Leslie Holmes
COSMOLOGY Peter Coles
CRIME FICTION Richard Bradford
CRIMINAL JUSTICE Julian V. Roberts
CRIMINOLOGY Tim Newburn
CRITICAL THEORY Stephen Eric Bronner
THE CRUSADES Christopher Tyerman
CRYPTOGRAPHY Fred Piper and Sean Murphy
CRYSTALLOGRAPHY A. M. Glazer
THE CULTURAL REVOLUTION Richard Curt Kraus
DADA AND SURREALISM David Hopkins
DANTE Peter Hainsworth and David Robey
DARWIN Jonathan Howard
THE DEAD SEA SCROLLS Timothy H. Lim
DECOLONIZATION Dane Kennedy
DEMOCRACY Bernard Crick
DEMOGRAPHY Sarah Harper
DEPRESSION Jan Scott and Mary Jane Tacchi
DERRIDA Simon Glendinning
DESCARTES Tom Sorell
DESERTS Nick Middleton
DESIGN John Heskett
DEVELOPMENT Ian Goldin
DEVELOPMENTAL BIOLOGY Lewis Wolpert
THE DEVIL Darren Oldridge
DIASPORA Kevin Kenny
DICTIONARIES Lynda Mugglestone
DINOSAURS David Norman
DIPLOMACY Joseph M. Siracusa
DOCUMENTARY FILM Patricia Aufderheide
DREAMING J. Allan Hobson
DRUGS Les Iversen
DRUIDS Barry Cunliffe
EARLY MUSIC Thomas Forrest Kelly
THE EARTH Martin Redfern
EARTH SYSTEM SCIENCE Tim Lenton
ECONOMICS Partha Dasgupta
EDUCATION Gary Thomas
EGYPTIAN MYTH Geraldine Pinch
EIGHTEENTH-CENTURY BRITAIN Paul Langford
THE ELEMENTS Philip Ball
EMOTION Dylan Evans
EMPIRE Stephen Howe
ENGELS Terrell Carver
ENGINEERING David Blockley
THE ENGLISH LANGUAGE Simon Horobin
ENGLISH LITERATURE Jonathan Bate
THE ENLIGHTENMENT John Robertson
ENTREPRENEURSHIP Paul Westhead and Mike Wright
ENVIRONMENTAL ECONOMICS Stephen Smith
ENVIRONMENTAL LAW Elizabeth Fisher
ENVIRONMENTAL POLITICS Andrew Dobson
EPICUREANISM Catherine Wilson
EPIDEMIOLOGY Rodolfo Saracci
ETHICS Simon Blackburn
ETHNOMUSICOLOGY Timothy Rice
THE ETRUSCANS Christopher Smith
EUGENICS Philippa Levine

THE EUROPEAN UNION
Simon Usherwood and John Pinder
EUROPEAN UNION LAW
Anthony Arnull
EVOLUTION Brian and
Deborah Charlesworth
EXISTENTIALISM Thomas Flynn
EXPLORATION Stewart A. Weaver
THE EYE Michael Land
FAIRY TALE Marina Warner
FAMILY LAW Jonathan Herring
FASCISM Kevin Passmore
FASHION Rebecca Arnold
FEMINISM Margaret Walters
FILM Michael Wood
FILM MUSIC Kathryn Kalinak
THE FIRST WORLD WAR
Michael Howard
FOLK MUSIC Mark Slobin
FOOD John Krebs
FORENSIC PSYCHOLOGY
David Canter
FORENSIC SCIENCE Jim Fraser
FORESTS Jaboury Ghazoul
FOSSILS Keith Thomson
FOUCAULT Gary Gutting
THE FOUNDING FATHERS
R. B. Bernstein
FRACTALS Kenneth Falconer
FREE SPEECH Nigel Warburton
FREE WILL Thomas Pink
FREEMASONRY Andreas Önnerfors
FRENCH LITERATURE John D. Lyons
THE FRENCH REVOLUTION
William Doyle
FREUD Anthony Storr
FUNDAMENTALISM Malise Ruthven
FUNGI Nicholas P. Money
THE FUTURE Jennifer M. Gidley
GALAXIES John Gribbin
GALILEO Stillman Drake
GAME THEORY Ken Binmore
GANDHI Bhikhu Parekh
GENES Jonathan Slack
GENIUS Andrew Robinson
GENOMICS John Archibald
GEOGRAPHY John Matthews
and David Herbert
GEOLOGY Jan Zalasiewicz
GEOPHYSICS William Lowrie
GEOPOLITICS Klaus Dodds
GERMAN LITERATURE Nicholas Boyle
GERMAN PHILOSOPHY
Andrew Bowie
GLOBAL CATASTROPHES Bill McGuire
GLOBAL ECONOMIC HISTORY
Robert C. Allen
GLOBALIZATION Manfred Steger
GOD John Bowker
GOETHE Ritchie Robertson
THE GOTHIC Nick Groom
GOVERNANCE Mark Bevir
GRAVITY Timothy Clifton
THE GREAT DEPRESSION AND
THE NEW DEAL Eric Rauchway
HABERMAS James Gordon Finlayson
THE HABSBURG EMPIRE
Martyn Rady
HAPPINESS Daniel M. Haybron
THE HARLEM RENAISSANCE
Cheryl A. Wall
THE HEBREW BIBLE AS LITERATURE
Tod Linafelt
HEGEL Peter Singer
HEIDEGGER Michael Inwood
THE HELLENISTIC AGE
Peter Thonemann
HEREDITY John Waller
HERMENEUTICS Jens Zimmermann
HERODOTUS Jennifer T. Roberts
HIEROGLYPHS Penelope Wilson
HINDUISM Kim Knott
HISTORY John H. Arnold
THE HISTORY OF ASTRONOMY
Michael Hoskin
THE HISTORY OF CHEMISTRY
William H. Brock
THE HISTORY OF CINEMA
Geoffrey Nowell-Smith
THE HISTORY OF LIFE
Michael Benton
THE HISTORY OF MATHEMATICS
Jacqueline Stedall
THE HISTORY OF MEDICINE
William Bynum
THE HISTORY OF PHYSICS
J. L. Heilbron
THE HISTORY OF TIME
Leofranc Holford-Strevens
HIV AND AIDS Alan Whiteside

HOBBES Richard Tuck
HOLLYWOOD Peter Decherney
THE HOLY ROMAN EMPIRE Joachim Whaley
HOME Michael Allen Fox
HORMONES Martin Luck
HUMAN ANATOMY Leslie Klenerman
HUMAN EVOLUTION Bernard Wood
HUMAN RIGHTS Andrew Clapham
HUMANISM Stephen Law
HUME A. J. Ayer
HUMOUR Noël Carroll
THE ICE AGE Jamie Woodward
IDEOLOGY Michael Freeden
THE IMMUNE SYSTEM Paul Klenerman
INDIAN CINEMA Ashish Rajadhyaksha
INDIAN PHILOSOPHY Sue Hamilton
THE INDUSTRIAL REVOLUTION Robert C. Allen
INFECTIOUS DISEASE Marta L. Wayne and Benjamin M. Bolker
INFINITY Ian Stewart
INFORMATION Luciano Floridi
INNOVATION Mark Dodgson and David Gann
INTELLIGENCE Ian J. Deary
INTELLECTUAL PROPERTY Siva Vaidhyanathan
INTERNATIONAL LAW Vaughan Lowe
INTERNATIONAL MIGRATION Khalid Koser
INTERNATIONAL RELATIONS Paul Wilkinson
INTERNATIONAL SECURITY Christopher S. Browning
IRAN Ali M. Ansari
ISLAM Malise Ruthven
ISLAMIC HISTORY Adam Silverstein
ISOTOPES Rob Ellam
ITALIAN LITERATURE Peter Hainsworth and David Robey
JESUS Richard Bauckham
JEWISH HISTORY David N. Myers
JOURNALISM Ian Hargreaves
JUDAISM Norman Solomon
JUNG Anthony Stevens
KABBALAH Joseph Dan
KAFKA Ritchie Robertson
KANT Roger Scruton
KEYNES Robert Skidelsky
KIERKEGAARD Patrick Gardiner
KNOWLEDGE Jennifer Nagel
THE KORAN Michael Cook
LAKES Warwick F. Vincent
LANDSCAPE ARCHITECTURE Ian H. Thompson
LANDSCAPES AND GEOMORPHOLOGY Andrew Goudie and Heather Viles
LANGUAGES Stephen R. Anderson
LATE ANTIQUITY Gillian Clark
LAW Raymond Wacks
THE LAWS OF THERMODYNAMICS Peter Atkins
LEADERSHIP Keith Grint
LEARNING Mark Haselgrove
LEIBNIZ Maria Rosa Antognazza
LIBERALISM Michael Freeden
LIGHT Ian Walmsley
LINCOLN Allen C. Guelzo
LINGUISTICS Peter Matthews
LITERARY THEORY Jonathan Culler
LOCKE John Dunn
LOGIC Graham Priest
LOVE Ronald de Sousa
MACHIAVELLI Quentin Skinner
MADNESS Andrew Scull
MAGIC Owen Davies
MAGNA CARTA Nicholas Vincent
MAGNETISM Stephen Blundell
MALTHUS Donald Winch
MAMMALS T. S. Kemp
MANAGEMENT John Hendry
MAO Delia Davin
MARINE BIOLOGY Philip V. Mladenov
THE MARQUIS DE SADE John Phillips
MARTIN LUTHER Scott H. Hendrix
MARTYRDOM Jolyon Mitchell
MARX Peter Singer
MATERIALS Christopher Hall
MATHEMATICS Timothy Gowers
THE MEANING OF LIFE Terry Eagleton
MEASUREMENT David Hand
MEDICAL ETHICS Tony Hope
MEDICAL LAW Charles Foster

MEDIEVAL BRITAIN John Gillingham and Ralph A. Griffiths
MEDIEVAL LITERATURE Elaine Treharne
MEDIEVAL PHILOSOPHY John Marenbon
MEMORY Jonathan K. Foster
METAPHYSICS Stephen Mumford
THE MEXICAN REVOLUTION Alan Knight
MICHAEL FARADAY Frank A. J. L. James
MICROBIOLOGY Nicholas P. Money
MICROECONOMICS Avinash Dixit
MICROSCOPY Terence Allen
THE MIDDLE AGES Miri Rubin
MILITARY JUSTICE Eugene R. Fidell
MILITARY STRATEGY Antulio J. Echevarria II
MINERALS David Vaughan
MIRACLES Yujin Nagasawa
MODERN ART David Cottington
MODERN CHINA Rana Mitter
MODERN DRAMA Kirsten E. Shepherd-Barr
MODERN FRANCE Vanessa R. Schwartz
MODERN INDIA Craig Jeffrey
MODERN IRELAND Senia Pašeta
MODERN ITALY Anna Cento Bull
MODERN JAPAN Christopher Goto-Jones
MODERN LATIN AMERICAN LITERATURE Roberto González Echevarría
MODERN WAR Richard English
MODERNISM Christopher Butler
MOLECULAR BIOLOGY Aysha Divan and Janice A. Royds
MOLECULES Philip Ball
MONASTICISM Stephen J. Davis
THE MONGOLS Morris Rossabi
MOONS David A. Rothery
MORMONISM Richard Lyman Bushman
MOUNTAINS Martin F. Price
MUHAMMAD Jonathan A. C. Brown
MULTICULTURALISM Ali Rattansi
MULTILINGUALISM John C. Maher
MUSIC Nicholas Cook
MYTH Robert A. Segal
THE NAPOLEONIC WARS Mike Rapport
NATIONALISM Steven Grosby
NATIVE AMERICAN LITERATURE Sean Teuton
NAVIGATION Jim Bennett
NELSON MANDELA Elleke Boehmer
NEOLIBERALISM Manfred Steger and Ravi Roy
NETWORKS Guido Caldarelli and Michele Catanzaro
THE NEW TESTAMENT Luke Timothy Johnson
THE NEW TESTAMENT AS LITERATURE Kyle Keefer
NEWTON Robert Iliffe
NIETZSCHE Michael Tanner
NINETEENTH-CENTURY BRITAIN Christopher Harvie and H. C. G. Matthew
THE NORMAN CONQUEST George Garnett
NORTH AMERICAN INDIANS Theda Perdue and Michael D. Green
NORTHERN IRELAND Marc Mulholland
NOTHING Frank Close
NUCLEAR PHYSICS Frank Close
NUCLEAR POWER Maxwell Irvine
NUCLEAR WEAPONS Joseph M. Siracusa
NUMBERS Peter M. Higgins
NUTRITION David A. Bender
OBJECTIVITY Stephen Gaukroger
OCEANS Dorrik Stow
THE OLD TESTAMENT Michael D. Coogan
THE ORCHESTRA D. Kern Holoman
ORGANIC CHEMISTRY Graham Patrick
ORGANIZED CRIME Georgios A. Antonopoulos and Georgios Papanicolaou
ORGANIZATIONS Mary Jo Hatch
PAGANISM Owen Davies
PAIN Rob Boddice
THE PALESTINIAN-ISRAELI CONFLICT Martin Bunton

PANDEMICS Christian W. McMillen
PARTICLE PHYSICS Frank Close
PAUL E. P. Sanders
PEACE Oliver P. Richmond
PENTECOSTALISM William K. Kay
PERCEPTION Brian Rogers
THE PERIODIC TABLE Eric R. Scerri
PHILOSOPHY Edward Craig
PHILOSOPHY IN THE ISLAMIC WORLD Peter Adamson
PHILOSOPHY OF LAW Raymond Wacks
PHILOSOPHY OF SCIENCE Samir Okasha
PHILOSOPHY OF RELIGION Tim Bayne
PHOTOGRAPHY Steve Edwards
PHYSICAL CHEMISTRY Peter Atkins
PILGRIMAGE Ian Reader
PLAGUE Paul Slack
PLANETS David A. Rothery
PLANTS Timothy Walker
PLATE TECTONICS Peter Molnar
PLATO Julia Annas
POLITICAL PHILOSOPHY David Miller
POLITICS Kenneth Minogue
POPULISM Cas Mudde and Cristóbal Rovira Kaltwasser
POSTCOLONIALISM Robert Young
POSTMODERNISM Christopher Butler
POSTSTRUCTURALISM Catherine Belsey
POVERTY Philip N. Jefferson
PREHISTORY Chris Gosden
PRESOCRATIC PHILOSOPHY Catherine Osborne
PRIVACY Raymond Wacks
PROBABILITY John Haigh
PROGRESSIVISM Walter Nugent
PROJECTS Andrew Davies
PROTESTANTISM Mark A. Noll
PSYCHIATRY Tom Burns
PSYCHOANALYSIS Daniel Pick
PSYCHOLOGY Gillian Butler and Freda McManus
PSYCHOLOGY OF MUSIC Elizabeth Hellmuth Margulis
PSYCHOTHERAPY Tom Burns and Eva Burns-Lundgren
PUBLIC ADMINISTRATION Stella Z. Theodoulou and Ravi K. Roy
PUBLIC HEALTH Virginia Berridge
PURITANISM Francis J. Bremer
THE QUAKERS Pink Dandelion
QUANTUM THEORY John Polkinghorne
RACISM Ali Rattansi
RADIOACTIVITY Claudio Tuniz
RASTAFARI Ennis B. Edmonds
THE REAGAN REVOLUTION Gil Troy
REALITY Jan Westerhoff
THE REFORMATION Peter Marshall
RELATIVITY Russell Stannard
RELIGION IN AMERICA Timothy Beal
THE RENAISSANCE Jerry Brotton
RENAISSANCE ART Geraldine A. Johnson
REVOLUTIONS Jack A. Goldstone
RHETORIC Richard Toye
RISK Baruch Fischhoff and John Kadvany
RITUAL Barry Stephenson
RIVERS Nick Middleton
ROBOTICS Alan Winfield
ROCKS Jan Zalasiewicz
ROMAN BRITAIN Peter Salway
THE ROMAN EMPIRE Christopher Kelly
THE ROMAN REPUBLIC David M. Gwynn
ROMANTICISM Michael Ferber
ROUSSEAU Robert Wokler
RUSSELL A. C. Grayling
RUSSIAN HISTORY Geoffrey Hosking
RUSSIAN LITERATURE Catriona Kelly
THE RUSSIAN REVOLUTION S. A. Smith
THE SAINTS Simon Yarrow
SAVANNAS Peter A. Furley
SCHIZOPHRENIA Chris Frith and Eve Johnstone
SCHOPENHAUER Christopher Janaway
SCIENCE AND RELIGION Thomas Dixon
SCIENCE FICTION David Seed
THE SCIENTIFIC REVOLUTION Lawrence M. Principe
SCOTLAND Rab Houston

SEXUAL SELECTION Marlene Zuk and Leigh W. Simmons
SEXUALITY Véronique Mottier
SHAKESPEARE'S COMEDIES Bart van Es
SHAKESPEARE'S SONNETS AND POEMS Jonathan F. S. Post
SHAKESPEARE'S TRAGEDIES Stanley Wells
SIKHISM Eleanor Nesbitt
THE SILK ROAD James A. Millward
SLANG Jonathon Green
SLEEP Steven W. Lockley and Russell G. Foster
SOCIAL AND CULTURAL ANTHROPOLOGY John Monaghan and Peter Just
SOCIAL PSYCHOLOGY Richard J. Crisp
SOCIAL WORK Sally Holland and Jonathan Scourfield
SOCIALISM Michael Newman
SOCIOLINGUISTICS John Edwards
SOCIOLOGY Steve Bruce
SOCRATES C. C. W. Taylor
SOUND Mike Goldsmith
THE SOVIET UNION Stephen Lovell
THE SPANISH CIVIL WAR Helen Graham
SPANISH LITERATURE Jo Labanyi
SPINOZA Roger Scruton
SPIRITUALITY Philip Sheldrake
SPORT Mike Cronin
STARS Andrew King
STATISTICS David J. Hand
STEM CELLS Jonathan Slack
STOICISM Brad Inwood
STRUCTURAL ENGINEERING David Blockley
STUART BRITAIN John Morrill
SUPERCONDUCTIVITY Stephen Blundell
SYMMETRY Ian Stewart
SYNTHETIC BIOLOGY Jamie A. Davies
TAXATION Stephen Smith
TEETH Peter S. Ungar
TELESCOPES Geoff Cottrell
TERRORISM Charles Townshend
THEATRE Marvin Carlson
THEOLOGY David F. Ford
THINKING AND REASONING Jonathan St B. T. Evans
THOMAS AQUINAS Fergus Kerr
THOUGHT Tim Bayne
TIBETAN BUDDHISM Matthew T. Kapstein
TOCQUEVILLE Harvey C. Mansfield
TRAGEDY Adrian Poole
TRANSLATION Matthew Reynolds
THE TROJAN WAR Eric H. Cline
TRUST Katherine Hawley
THE TUDORS John Guy
TWENTIETH-CENTURY BRITAIN Kenneth O. Morgan
THE UNITED NATIONS Jussi M. Hanhimäki
THE U.S. CONGRESS Donald A. Ritchie
THE U.S. CONSTITUTION David J. Bodenhamer
THE U.S. SUPREME COURT Linda Greenhouse
UTILITARIANISM Katarzyna de Lazari-Radek and Peter Singer
UNIVERSITIES AND COLLEGES David Palfreyman and Paul Temple
UTOPIANISM Lyman Tower Sargent
VETERINARY SCIENCE James Yeates
THE VIKINGS Julian Richards
VIRUSES Dorothy H. Crawford
VOLTAIRE Nicholas Cronk
WAR AND TECHNOLOGY Alex Roland
WATER John Finney
WEATHER Storm Dunlop
THE WELFARE STATE David Garland
WILLIAM SHAKESPEARE Stanley Wells
WITCHCRAFT Malcolm Gaskill
WITTGENSTEIN A. C. Grayling
WORK Stephen Fineman
WORLD MUSIC Philip Bohlman
THE WORLD TRADE ORGANIZATION Amrita Narlikar
WORLD WAR II Gerhard L. Weinberg
WRITING AND SCRIPT Andrew Robinson
ZIONISM Michael Stanislawski

Available soon:

MODERN ARCHITECTURE Adam Sharr
BIOMETRICS Michael Fairhurst
GLACIATION David J. A. Evans
TYPOGRAPHY Paul Luna
ENVIRONMENTAL ETHICS Robin Attfield

For more information visit our website

www.oup.com/vsi/

Tom Burns

PSYCHIATRY

A Very Short Introduction

SECOND EDITION

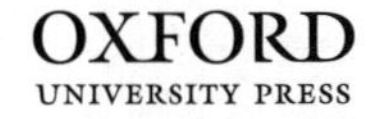

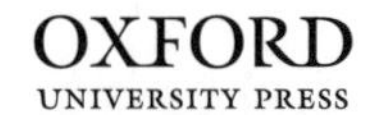

Great Clarendon Street, Oxford, OX2 6DP,
United Kingdom

Oxford University Press is a department of the University of Oxford.
It furthers the University's objective of excellence in research, scholarship,
and education by publishing worldwide. Oxford is a registered trade mark of
Oxford University Press in the UK and in certain other countries

First edition published 2006
Second edition published 2018

Impression: 1

Published in the United States of America by Oxford University Press
198 Madison Avenue, New York, NY 10016, United States of America

British Library Cataloguing in Publication Data
Data available

Library of Congress Control Number: 2018944719

ISBN 978-0-19-882620-0

Printed in Great Britain by
Ashford Colour Press Ltd, Gosport, Hampshire

Contents

Preface

Psychiatry currently insists that it is 'just another branch of medicine', like cardiology or oncology. This emphasis has two aims. First, to make psychiatry more respectable as a profession. By highlighting its scientific credentials, its commitment to precise diagnoses and evidence-based treatments, it increases its status within medicine and in society generally. Second, to reduce the stigma which has always been associated with mental illnesses. Stressing that they are illnesses like any other illness ('mental illnesses are brain diseases') aims to reduce the prejudice experienced by sufferers and the sense of responsibility and shame felt by so many patients and families. We don't feel ashamed or blame ourselves if a family member develops arthritis, so why do we if they become depressed? It is against this backdrop of unnecessary additional suffering that psychiatry's medical legitimacy is, quite rightly, stressed.

But it is not that simple. Psychiatry *is* different. Even those of us who work in it are treated as different. I am often asked, only half-joking, whether we become psychiatrists because we are odd or do we become odd by being psychiatrists. The *New Yorker Magazine* produces a separate compilation of psychiatrist cartoons because they print so many.

Psychiatry can also inspire fear. Its doctors are, after all, the only ones who can legally compel treatment. Special laws exist in all developed countries, both to protect the mentally ill against punishment but also if necessary to compel treatment. There is a remarkable international consensus about the reality and importance of mental illnesses despite, as we will observe, the absence of simple objective definitions of them.

There is also a fascination about psychiatry that goes beyond the natural curiosity about how the body or mind works. Psychoanalysts have suggested that this fascination (often mixed with fear) is because mental illnesses act out our own inner dramas. We see the depression we are struggling with and containing displayed before us, or individuals losing control when we may fear (or secretly long) to let go and shed our inhibitions.

There is certainly some truth in this. As explored in Chapter 1 the illnesses psychiatry deals with are diagnosed on the basis of experiences and feelings which are familiar to us all. Yet they convey a sense of 'difference' at the same time. We identify with the descriptions, yet recognize that some important threshold has been crossed. Psychiatry's increasing scientific sophistication has sharpened that threshold with enormous advances in consistency of diagnosis. However, Chapter 6 outlines some undesired consequences of this increased certainty.

Psychiatry is, like all medicine, a pragmatic problem-solving activity. It draws on scientific theories but it is not derived from theories or limited by them. Unlike psychology or physics, psychiatry cannot be derived 'top-down' from basic principles. Psychiatry has been formed by the illnesses that it has been required (and agreed) to treat and been further shaped by the treatments it had available at the time. Chapter 1 includes descriptions of schizophrenia and manic depression and how these diseases moulded the fledgling profession. Psychiatry's development reflects the values and structures of the societies that foster it. It is almost impossible to understand current practices without some understanding of that history which is covered in Chapters 2 and 3. Similarly, the now relatively neglected contribution of psychoanalysis and psychotherapy is addressed in Chapter 4.

Chapters 5 and 6 deal with the controversies that have raged around and within psychiatry ever since it first emerged as a profession. It is a fair criticism of this book that it devotes more space to these controversies than to psychiatry's undeniable advances. I could have dwelt more on new drugs, improved psychological treatments, and working practices which have contributed enormously to human welfare. Psychiatry and the neurosciences are making remarkable strides.

I have dwelt on the controversial aspects of psychiatry for two reasons. First, because they demonstrate real philosophical and ethical differences between mental and physical illnesses which won't go away. Technological advances will not obliterate these tensions; rather, as explored in Chapters 6 and 7, more effective treatments often sharpen them. The challenge for psychiatry in the 21st century may be particularly acute in the ethical and social questions posed by increasingly sophisticated and powerful treatments of the mind. Second, psychiatry is the arena where many of the big questions of the time—philosophical, political, and social—have to be hammered out on the anvil of real human relations and suffering. The philosophical debate about free will and determinism comes alive in the courtroom arguments over a psychiatric defence or in government policy about the management of psychopaths. The politics of power and social control drove the dismantling of the asylums and now frames the debate on compulsory treatment. The mind–brain dichotomy hovers throughout. The sustained battering from the anti-psychiatrists in the 1960s and 1970s (Chapter 5) raised the right (indeed, they would say the existential *obligation*) to be different.

So, welcome to an area of medicine that is both mysterious and exciting as advances in brain sciences continually bump up against the messy reality of human beings. Psychiatry is an activity which, despite the scanners and designer drugs, still rests on establishing trusting personal relationships. And lastly, welcome to a pursuit that keeps challenging us about what it is to be truly human; continually reminding us of those unresolved philosophical issues (free will, mind–body dualism, personal autonomy versus social obligations) that we usually push to the back of our minds in order to simply get on with life.

List of illustrations

The publisher and the author apologize for any errors or omissions in this list. If contacted they will be pleased to rectify these at the earliest opportunity.

Chapter 1
What is psychiatry?

The only normal people are the ones you don't know very well.

All of us know someone who is troubled (anxious, depressed, or confused) and most of us have felt that way ourselves at some time. At such times our emotions may be overwhelming and difficult to control and our thoughts strange and bizarre. The media don't help by repeating exaggerated claims that one in four of us 'has a mental health disorder' or that a fifth of students are suffering from 'mental health issues'.

Does this mean that we have been mentally ill or need to see a psychiatrist? Luckily, the answer for most of us is no. Yet when we read about psychiatry what we find described are experiences remarkably similar to our own. Psychiatry is fascinating because it deals with consciousness, choice, motivation, free will, relationships—indeed everything that makes us human. While it is often cloaked in forbidding jargon ('affect' instead of mood, 'anxiety' instead of worry, 'phobia' rather than fear, 'cognition' instead of thinking), the conditions described are still instantly recognizable.

This is the persisting paradox about psychiatry that will recur throughout this book—that its subject is simultaneously firmly rooted in common human experience and yet is somehow 'that bit different'. Patients' experiences are immediately familiar to us, yet they are used to diagnose disorders quite outside our experience. Hopefully by the end of this book you will understand this dilemma better, but I cannot promise to resolve it for you. It's been argued about since psychiatry came into being and the argument still goes on. However, it may be best to start by defining what psychiatry is (and what it is not), before returning to the philosophical and political controversies that attend it.

All the 'psychs': psychology, psychotherapy, psychoanalysis, and psychiatry

'Psyche' is the Greek word for mind. These four terms describe different approaches to understanding and helping individuals with psychological and emotional (mental) problems. There is lots of overlap, and sometimes the same individual can describe herself using more than one of them, so it is not surprising that people get confused. Getting the differences clear will help clarify what psychiatry is.

Psychology

Psychology is the study of thought and behaviour. It originated just over a century ago from a tradition of introspective philosophy (trying to understand the minds of others by understanding your own) and is now a firmly established science. It includes the study and understanding of mental processes in all their aspects and it has many branches. *Experimental psychologists* conduct careful experiments to explore mental functioning (perception, memory, arousal, risk-taking, etc.). They do not restrict themselves exclusively to humans but study animals both in their own right and as models for human behaviour. Experimental psychology is generally considered a 'hard science' and follows the same rigorous principles of investigation as physics or chemistry.

There are several professions within psychology (e.g. *educational psychologists, industrial psychologists, forensic psychologists*). *Clinical psychologists* have postgraduate training in abnormal psychology to help people deal with their problems. Their first approaches used learning theory (i.e. consistent rewards and punishments to shape behaviour) in behaviour therapy. This was particularly successful in helping disturbed children and those with learning difficulties to modify their behaviour. Its great strength is that it works directly without the patient needing to understand it. Psychological treatments are now much more sophisticated and one of the most successful and widely practised psychotherapies (cognitive behaviour therapy) has been developed and provided mainly by clinical psychologists who are now essential members of all modern mental health ('psychiatric') services.

Psychoanalysis

Psychoanalysis is the method of treating neurotic disorders developed by Sigmund Freud towards the end of the 19th century in Vienna. In psychoanalysis the patient is encouraged to relax and say the first thing that comes into their mind ('free association') and to pay close attention to their dreams and to their 'irrational' thoughts. Freud believed that neuroses arose because patients tried to keep unconscious ('repress') thoughts and feelings that were unacceptable to them. The analyst listens carefully and detects patterns which are clues to these 'conflicts'. By sharing these insights ('interpretations') he or she helps patients confront and resolve them. Psychoanalysis is intensive, traditionally with five one-hour sessions a week for several years. Psychoanalysis is the origin of the cartoon image of the bearded psychiatrist sitting behind the patient lying on a couch.

Although Freud was a doctor, psychoanalysts do not need to be medically qualified. In the Americas (where psychoanalysis has been most influential) analysts were usually also psychiatrists, but this is increasingly the exception. Analysts rarely use their medical knowledge—they make a virtue of not 'interfering' beyond the analysis. There are several schools of psychoanalysis developed by disciples of Freud (e.g. Jung, Adler, Klein) and some have become quite remote from the original model (e.g. Reich, Lacan). Psychoanalysis has had enormous influence beyond psychiatry. Terms like 'Freudian' and 'Freudian slip' are part of everyday speech. It remains highly revered and influential in the arts and social studies but, because of limited scientific evidence of its efficacy, is increasingly marginalized in modern psychiatry.

Psychotherapy

It soon became obvious that there was more to psychoanalysis than Freud's original remote and neutral exploration of the unconscious. The relationships formed in this intense treatment were very powerful and analysts began to explore them experimenting with more active and varied therapies (time-limited, structured forms, therapies in groups, therapies in families, etc.). These psychological approaches, in which the relationship is used actively through talking to promote self-awareness and change, are broadly understood as 'psychotherapy'. Most early psychotherapies relied heavily on Freud's theories and are called 'psychodynamic' to emphasize the impact of thoughts and feelings over time. Several of the newer ones draw on a wider range of theoretical backgrounds and their varied forms are dealt with in greater detail in *Psychotherapy: A Very Short Introduction.*

What they all have in common is that they use communication within a formalized and secure relationship to explore difficulties and find ways of either adapting to them or overcoming them. Most psychodynamic psychotherapies also require (like psychoanalysis) that the therapist undergoes a treatment themselves as part of the training. Becoming a psychoanalyst remains very tightly controlled, but psychotherapy is generally less formal. Some schools of psychotherapy are strict about whom they admit but the title 'psychotherapist' could, until recently, be used by anyone. Most psychotherapists are not psychiatrists and, sadly, psychotherapy skills are much less central to psychiatry training than previously, although there are some psychiatrists who work mainly as psychotherapists. Chapter 4 is devoted to psychoanalysis and psychotherapy.

What is psychiatry?

So if it is not psychology nor psychoanalysis nor psychotherapy, what is psychiatry? There are overlaps with the other 'psychs' but there are some fundamental differences. First and foremost psychiatry is a branch of *medicine*—you cannot become a psychiatrist without first qualifying as a doctor. Having qualified, the future psychiatrist spends several years in further training. Your psychiatrist is increasingly likely to be a woman. Half of newly qualified doctors are women and they are more likely than men to enter psychiatry. This is for a variety of reasons ranging from work/life balance to a greater ease with the relational aspects of the role. She then works with, and learns about, mental illnesses in exactly the same way that a dermatologist would train by treating patients with skin disorders or an obstetrician by delivering babies. Within medicine, psychiatry is simply defined as that branch which deals with 'mental illnesses' (nowadays often called 'psychiatric disorders').

Medicine is fundamentally a pragmatic practice. It draws heavily on biological sciences and scientific methods, but the ultimate test of a treatment is if the patient gets better. We don't have to know *how* the treatment works, just *if* it works. So psychiatry is not based on theory, as in psychology or psychoanalysis, but on practice. Whatever is viewed as a mental illness (and this has changed over time), and whatever treatments are available for these illnesses, will determine what psychiatry is.

What is a mental illness?

There is a marked circularity about this ('a psychiatrist is someone who diagnoses and treats psychiatric disorders', 'psychiatric disorders are those conditions which are diagnosed and treated by psychiatrists'). There has been endless controversy about the reliability of psychiatric diagnoses and even whether or not mental illnesses exist at all (Chapter 5). It is worth spending a little time on why psychiatric diagnoses are so controversial because the question keeps cropping up (despite the same issues applying across medicine).

The subjectivity of diagnosis

The hallmark of the psychiatrist's trade is the interview. We make our diagnoses (and still conduct most of our treatment) in face-to-face discussions with patients. We take a careful history (as do all doctors), but then, instead of conducting a physical examination (feeling the abdomen, taking the pulse, listening through a stethoscope), we conduct what is called a 'mental state exam'. In this we probe deeper into what is worrying the patient, their mood, ways of thinking, etc. Some of this involves simply noting what the patient has reported (that they are hearing strange sounds or that they panic every time they think of going out). Psychiatrists try to go beyond this and try to get a sense of the patient's world, understanding what they are going through. This process aims to go beyond listing symptoms and to record 'phenomenology' (giving an insight into the patient's experience). It requires 'directed empathy', actively using the psychiatrist's own responses in the interview to understand what the patient is feeling and thinking, even if this is not expressed in words. For instance we may conclude that a patient recounting a series of vindictive acts from strangers and friends alike is, in fact, over-aroused and misinterpreting innocent events.

This ability to grasp how other people experience things and what they are feeling is an essential human capacity. Understanding how others see the world from their perspective is called having 'a theory of mind'. It is so highly developed we can manage up to four levels ('I understand how he understands his (other) view of her understanding…etc.…'). It is so necessary that its absence, as in autism or Asperger's Syndrome, is a profound handicap. Psychiatrists train this skill and, because of increasing familiarity with the range of common disorders, can use it actively to understand the confused and confusing experiences that patients recount.

Psychiatric diagnoses do not depend on physical indicators—there are no blood tests or X-rays. A written list of what is said or a detailed description of the behaviour (e.g. recording the diagnostic criteria for depression) are only part of the process. Psychiatric diagnoses rely on a judgement about *why* someone is doing something, not just the observation of *what* they are doing. Hence the criticism that they are not scientific or 'objective'. A profoundly depressed elderly man may not say that he is depressed but instead complain of tiredness, aches and pains, poor sleep, and feelings of guilt. Indeed he might not speak at all. A psychiatrist will probably understand this immobility as depressive. She concludes that this is a result of despair and hopelessness rather than because of a wide range of possible physical causes.

Imposing categories on dimensions

We cherish human variation. We would hate a world where everyone had the same personality, no over-sensitive individuals, no moody individuals, no brave or brash ones. Similarly life without emotional variation would be intolerable. Aldous Huxley's book *Brave New World* (where everyone remained constantly content by taking a drug called 'Soma') was a dystopia, not a utopia. Normal intensities of sadness as in grief, or fear as in a house fire, match anything in mental illnesses. There is no consistent cut-off, no absolute distinction between the normal and the abnormal. Even hearing voices when there is nobody about (auditory hallucinations) occurs in perfectly 'normal' people. Widows and widowers regularly hear the voice of their dead partner quite clearly and usually find it comforting. So why do psychiatrists list hallucinations as symptoms of mental illness?

Medical practice involves pattern recognition. For most disorders there is a set of symptoms and signs that characterize it. Not all have to be present to make the diagnosis, although obviously that makes it easier. If some of the symptoms are very prominent then we hardly need to confirm the others, but if none is very striking we will seek to complete the picture. The intensity and duration of the symptoms also matter (how long the anxiety lasts, how persistent and disruptive the voices). Judgements must also accommodate cultural differences. Northern Europeans are usually considered less emotionally demonstrative than southern Europeans; expressions of distress differ, for example, between a Finn and an Italian.

Traditionally medical training involved seeing as many patients as possible to learn these patterns within the range of human variation. Recently diagnostic systems have become more formalized, insisting on the presence of some key features and then a selection of others. The current diagnostic criteria for depression used in ICD-10 (International Classification of Diseases) and DSM5 (Diagnostic and Statistical Manual (of the American Psychiatric Association)) are examples. These systems require the psychiatrist to decide if one or two core features are present. These have certainly improved consistency, but the process is still the same. In DSM5 either 'depressed mood' or 'loss of interest or pleasure' must be present for at least two weeks plus four other symptoms such as weight loss, insomnia, fatigue, agitation, etc. out of a list of nine. In addition the symptoms must be judged to cause significant distress or impairment of social function and not be due to an identified medical condition.

Depression is treated as a yes/no, present/absent quality, when we all know that mood varies continuously between people and over time. Psychiatric diagnoses require the imposition of *categories* (yes/no, present/absent) onto what are really *dimensions* (a little/ quite a bit/a bit more/quite a lot/too much) and this is down to professional judgement.

This is very obvious in psychiatry, but it is certainly not unique to it. Our popular view of illnesses is usually based on the examples of infectious diseases or surgical trauma—you've either got measles or not, your leg is either broken or not. There is no ambiguity and no need to establish consensus. However, few illnesses are that straightforward. Even the infection example is not that simple—you can find the same bacteria that cause pneumonia in the lungs of perfectly healthy people. The diagnosis is not made just by finding the bacteria but by finding them in the presence of a fever and cough. Even objective, verifiable data don't always resolve the issue. What is considered 'pathological' will change depending on changing knowledge about diseases and available treatments. Just as improved treatments have led us to lower the threshold for depression, so the diagnosis of disorders as apparently concrete and measurable as diabetes and high blood pressure is constantly redefined.

So psychiatry is not for the faint-hearted or those who crave too much intellectual security. It is, of all the branches of medicine, the one that most clearly exposes the processes behind making a diagnosis. The language is revealing—doctors 'make' diagnoses, they impose patterns rather than simply discovering them. It is also the branch of medicine which most explicitly recognizes the impact of individual history and personality on its practice. Both the definitions of disorders used by psychiatrists and their expression in individuals are moulded by our expectations. We now identify and treat battle stress or shell shock in war as a psychiatric disorder, whereas a century ago we punished it as cowardice. Young adults in the 21st century will seek help for problems in a manner utterly unrecognizable to how their stoical grandparents would have behaved. This doesn't make psychiatry particularly unscientific or unreliable (psychiatric diagnoses are about as reliable as those in medicine overall). However, it reminds us that, like all medicine, it remains (despite wishful thinking) still as much an art as a science and draws from both the social and physical sciences.

The scope of psychiatry—psychoses, neuroses, and personality problems

Psychiatrists deal with a wide range of problems. The most severe disorders are often referred to as 'functional' (or non-organic) psychoses and include schizophrenia and manic depression (now called bipolar disorder). The distinction into organic and non-organic is rather messy but still useful. Although we are increasingly convinced that there are organic (usually brain) changes underlying many of these illnesses, 'organic' is reserved for those psychoses arising from another, usually very obvious, disease, such as head injury, and dementia or severe infections. Functional psychoses are the conditions to which the older term 'madness' was applied. The 'function' of the brain is disordered, not its structure. Overall they affect about 3 per cent of the population at some stage in their life. So while they are not very common neither are they that rare—about one person in an average secondary school class will suffer a psychotic illness in the course of their adult life.

A striking characteristic of psychosis is the loss of insight into the origins of the current strange experiences. The patient loses the ability to 'reality test'—to check his or her terrifying or melancholic thoughts and feelings against what is really going on. He cannot think, 'I'm blaming myself for everything and cannot see a way forward because I'm depressed.' Rather, he thinks, 'I feel this way as punishment for what I've done and there is no future.' He may actively deny that he is ill and resist the attempts of those around him to balance these misinterpretations. Being so fixated on internal experiences, unable to modify them despite evidence to the contrary, is loosely referred to as lacking insight. The patient denies that he is ill and cannot recognize that family or mental health staff want to help. Psychoses can be terrifying experiences generating high levels of anxiety and distress. The two major psychoses have so shaped psychiatry that they deserve detailed consideration.

Schizophrenia

Schizophrenia is our usual image of severe mental illnesses. It does not mean split personality—Dr Jekyll and Mr Hyde was not a case of schizophrenia. The name was introduced by a Swiss doctor, Eugen Bleuler, in 1911 to emphasize the disintegration ('splitting') of mental functioning. It will affect just under 1 per cent of the population worldwide and usually starts in early adulthood (during the twenties) although it can occur earlier or later. Men and women are equally affected but men often become ill earlier and fare worse. The obvious features are hallucinations, delusions, disordered thinking, social withdrawal, and self-neglect. A current theory of schizophrenia emphasizes a disorder of 'salience'—being unable to distinguish figure from background. Hence the failure to distinguish internal drives from external events.

Hallucinations are 'sensory experiences without stimuli'. Far and away the most common are auditory hallucinations—hearing voices which talk to the patient or talk about them. Seeing things is not uncommon (though rarely as complete or persistent as auditory hallucinations) and many patients describe strange physical sensations in their body. Hallucinations are not simply imagining our thoughts as a voice in the head—most of us do that. They are experienced with the full force of an external event, fully awake and in broad daylight; there is no 'as if' quality to them and the patient believes they are absolutely real.

Delusions are 'firm, fixed false ideas that are inconsistent with the patient's culture or experience'. Deciding that something is a delusion requires more understanding of context than identifying a hallucination. The striking thing about delusions is the *intensity* with which they are held and how impervious they are to argument or proof to the contrary. The patient has no doubt whatever about their truth and importance.

We live increasingly in a multi-cultural society and it can be difficult to decide whether an idea really is that odd for any particular individual. For example, two quite different patients described to me their conviction that there were invisible force fields criss-crossing their living rooms which they experienced vividly. The first was a young woman preoccupied with Ley lines, Druidic culture, and Eastern mysticism. No illness here. The second was a retired schoolmistress who was convinced the force fields were electric, originated from her neighbour, and represented an attempt to influence her sexually. This latter is a classic delusion in late-onset schizophrenia and caused her to rip out the electrical wiring in her house to get at its source. In schizophrenia delusions are commonly persecutory ('paranoid'), but the source of the persecution (e.g. police, communists, the devil, freemasons) varies across time and place.

Thought disorder as a symptom is often considered particularly characteristic of schizophrenia. Schizophrenia differs from other psychiatric disorders in that not only is the *content* of thought often unusual (not surprising given the impact of hallucinations and delusions), but its logical and grammatical *form* can be disturbed. With severe thought disorder it can sometimes be impossible to understand what the patient means, although each individual word can be understood. At its extreme, speech can be totally incomprehensible with lots of invented words and jumbled sentences. More often, however, while sentences appear logical they lead nowhere or cannot be recalled or understood.

Obviously you have to be careful before diagnosing thought disorder that it isn't just that the patient is cleverer than you or knows more (both always a possibility). However, recovered patients often tell us that at these times they did not feel fully in control of their thoughts. They may have experienced thoughts being directly inserted into, or withdrawn from, their minds or that they became suddenly aware of new connections between things that were uniquely revealed to them. This sense of *unique new meanings* is rare in other conditions and can lead to words being used in different and puzzling ways. A patient who had just 'become aware' that the colour green 'meant intimacy' (didn't imply intimacy, wasn't associated with intimacy, but *meant* intimacy) constructed sentences using it this way fully convinced that we also understood it.

Withdrawal and self-neglect are probably among the most distressing and disabling features of schizophrenia. Bleuler, who first used the term in 1911, thought that withdrawal from engagement with others was central to the disorder, and he used the term 'autism' to describe it. Although Bleuler coined the term schizophrenia, he was not the first to describe it. Kraepelin did that in 1896, but he called it 'dementia praecox' based on the gradual withdrawal and deterioration which he thought always occurred. Both these early researchers considered what we now call the 'positive symptoms' (hallucinations, delusions, and thought disorder) to be secondary to the core process of withdrawal and turning inward—now called 'negative symptoms'.

Since the development of antipsychotic drugs (which target these positive symptoms), we have tended to see it the other way round—that the negative symptoms are a consequence of the positive ones. After each acute episode patients did not get fully better, they were that bit less engaged, less interested in themselves or the world around them. However, the pendulum is swinging back with more attention to these negative symptoms, not least because our drug treatments are much less effective with them.

Kraepelin was very gloomy about schizophrenia and believed that virtually no patients really got fully better, but Bleuler was more positive, and current thinking lies closer to him. Schizophrenia is a fluctuating illness and most patients experience several relapses. About a quarter probably recover well, with just one or two episodes. Most, however, have several episodes and take longer to get better after each one, rarely achieving 100 per cent recovery. A small proportion of patients have a very poor outcome indeed and spend much of their adult lives unable to live independently. Modern treatments, particularly antipsychotic drugs, mean that most patients only come into hospital for a few weeks or months when they relapse, not the years that characterized pre-war mental hospitals. There is little real argument any longer that genetics play a role, though it is far from the only risk (see Chapter 5). There seems to have been a small reduction in the incidence of schizophrenia over the last century, although recent use of high-potency cannabis ('skunk') appears not only to precipitate relapses but to contribute to its onset.

Manic depressive disorder (bipolar disorder)

Modern psychiatric classification owes its intellectual origins to Kraepelin's distinction between schizophrenia and manic depressive illness. This is now renamed bipolar disorder, the term used from here on. In Kraepelin's time mental hospitals admitted whoever was sent to them; some got better but many didn't. There was not that much attention to diagnosis other than perhaps distinguishing the learning disabled and the epileptic from the psychotic. Kraepelin noted that one group of psychosis patients alternated through several discrete periods of profound disturbances—sometimes agitated and sometimes withdrawn and depressed. What distinguished them most, however, from the schizophrenia patients was that they made good recoveries between these episodes and more of them eventually left hospital. It was the *course* of the illness rather than its symptoms that impressed him (see Chapter 2).

Bipolar disorder is now the accepted term, but this is a significantly broader diagnosis than manic depression. Manic depressive patients *can* have all the same symptoms as in schizophrenia (hallucinations, delusions, thought disorder, etc.), although these occur only in the most severe forms of mania and depression. However, these symptoms are always accompanied by a disturbance of mood—either depression or elation. This elation is called mania (often softened to hypomania). In the depressed phase the patient suffers from severe depression and may be suicidal. In the elated phase they are overactive and bursting with confidence and energy. Hypomanic patients can be very destructive to themselves—spending money they haven't got and behaving in an uninhibited manner (drinking too much, being sexually overactive, short-tempered, driving too fast, etc.). The psychotic symptoms, where they occur, reflect the prevailing mood. If the patient is depressed hallucinations will be critical and persecuting, if elated the hallucinations praise and encourage. Depressive delusions are usually of guilt and worthlessness and hypomanic delusions are expansive and grandiose: 'I'm going to be asked to advise the president about foreign policy', 'My paintings are worth millions.'

In less extreme forms of hypomania patients can be very entertaining, often talking fast ('pressure of speech'), punning, and making humorous associations ('flight of ideas'). Many famous entertainers and artists have suffered from bipolar disorder and acknowledge that they get their inspiration when they are 'high'. It can be difficult to be certain about diagnosis in some of the milder forms of hypomania because it usually lacks the 'strangeness' of the schizophrenic episode. The main disturbance is one of judgement—we all wish we were richer or hope that our paintings are brilliant, but we usually know better. Often the diagnosis needs friends and family members to be able to confirm that this is not just how the patient usually is.

A rather flamboyant, flirty TV executive was brought to the clinic by her worried mother. The story was not, in itself, that remarkable—some rather torrid love affairs with work colleagues, recreational drug use in night clubs, and some rudeness to her boss and absences from work. There are lots of creative people who conduct their lives like this. What was decisive was her mother's description of how normally she was an over-conscientious, rather anxious woman and that this was completely out of character. The mother was alert to the issue because her late husband was bipolar.

Like schizophrenia, manic depression also affects just under 1 per cent of the population although bipolar disorder has been diagnosed in up to 3 per cent. It also runs in families, starts in early adult life (though usually later than schizophrenia), and males and females are affected about equally. Although the elated phases are more dramatic, depression is more frequent and persistent. The depressive phase of bipolar disorder is not easily distinguishable from the more common clinical depression.

Treatment of psychotic disorders

This is not a book to deal in any detail with individual treatments. Treatments in psychiatry, like any other branch of medicine, are evolving fast so any description here would soon be out of date.

A range of drugs have been developed since the 1950s ('antipsychotics' such as chlorpromazine, haloperidol, risperidone, clozapine, olanzapine) which are effective in settling patients during the acute phases of psychosis. These tranquillizing drugs calm the mind without making the patient fall asleep, as earlier sedatives did. Antipsychotics have revolutionized the treatment of acute psychotic episodes with calmer, shorter spells in hospital. Continuing on antipsychotics after recovery reduces the risk of further breakdowns, and most psychiatrists encourage schizophrenia patients to stay on them for many, many years ('maintenance treatment'). Obviously this is not easy as all drugs have side effects and nobody likes taking them endlessly. With support, however, many patients do succeed in staying on them and suffer far fewer breakdowns.

Severe depressive episodes in bipolar patients can be treated either with antidepressants or, in extreme cases, with the ever-controversial electro-convulsive treatment (ECT). These are discussed in Chapters 2 and 3. There are also now a number of 'mood stabilizers' such as lithium or sodium valproate which are used in the maintenance treatment of bipolar disorder and significantly reduce the risk of breakdown. Drugs are certainly not the only treatments available for psychotic disorders (Chapter 3), but they are currently the cornerstone.

Compulsory treatment

Lack of insight can pose real risks of a psychotic patient harming himself or others as he tries to flee or defend himself from perceived threats or persecution. Because of this loss of insight, and the risks posed during psychotic states, psychiatry has been unique within medicine in that the patient's right to refuse treatment can be overruled. This is dealt with in more detail in Chapters 2 and 6. Provision for some compulsory treatment is universal in psychiatric services and widely accepted. The conditions under which it can be applied, however (who imposes it, whether it is restricted to hospital care, whether there needs to be immediate risk of physical danger, etc.), vary enormously from country to country.

Compulsory detention for the severely mentally ill evolved before there were any effective treatments. It arose from a recognition that mental illness is not simply deviance ('mad' not 'bad'). In mental illnesses the individual was changed from his normal self, and could change back. Detaining the patient served to protect him or her while the illness ran its course, until they recovered. Sadly, not everyone does get better, but enough do to sustain the humanitarian impulse behind detention.

Depression and neurotic disorders

Not all psychiatric disorders involve the break with reality found in psychoses. In fact the majority of patients seen by psychiatrists do not suffer from psychoses but from less devastating disorders. Most of these are characterized by high levels of depression and anxiety. They used to be lumped together under the title of 'neuroses', but the term has become unfashionable in psychiatry. However, it is a useful term, albeit rather vague, and one that most people understand, so it will be used here. Neuroses cause distress and suffering to those who have them but may not be obvious to others. They vary greatly in severity. Most patients are able to lead normal lives (marrying and working) while coping with them, but some can be as disabling as psychoses.

Depression

Depression is the commonest psychiatric disorder and affects about 15 per cent of us in our lifetime. The World Health Organization ranks it second to heart disease as a cause of disability worldwide. It appears to be becoming more common (particularly in the developed world), although some of this may be better detection, greater public awareness, and greater willingness to seek help. Luckily, with the advent of antidepressants and the development of more effective psychological treatments (e.g. cognitive behaviour therapy), it usually gets better fairly quickly. With treatment over two-thirds of patients are recovered by six months, and with milder depressions a third recover in this time even without treatment. The effectiveness of antidepressants has recently been challenged, but the weight of evidence is that they do work in all but the most mild cases and roughly double the rate of recovery. Most patients are treated by their family doctor and only the most severe get referred to psychiatrists. A proportion of depressed patients eventually become diagnosed as having bipolar disorder, but here we focus on the 'non-psychotic' group.

Depression is usually experienced as a profound sense of misery, a loss of hope, often with self-doubt and self-criticism. Tension and anxiety are very common, sleep is disturbed, and patients lose weight and find themselves unable to concentrate properly or get on with things. Tearfulness and thoughts of suicide are common and aches, pains, and health worries frequent. In more severe cases patients report 'feeling nothing' (being cold and empty, unable to enjoy anything) rather than sadness. Patients may also take to alcohol or drugs as self-medication, which invariably makes things worse. Depression differs from our normal periods of sadness by having a life of its own, going on and on without relief, entrenched by the weight loss and poor sleep.

Depression is three times more common in women than men. Some people are constitutionally or temperamentally more at risk of developing it, but it is clearly influenced by life circumstances. It is much more common in those living in poverty, those who are unemployed, live alone, have few friends, or who have painful or disabling physical illnesses. Early loss of a mother and a difficult or abusive childhood are associated with an increased risk of becoming depressed as an adult. Depression is also more likely to follow from severe personal problems (relationship break-ups, exam failure, job loss, etc.).

Helping people with depression almost always needs more than antidepressants (though these are very effective). Counselling, help to see a way forward, specific psychotherapy, a supportive social network, and help building resilience are all needed. Understanding depression better has led to the recognition of just how important social networks and friendships are to people. These are not optional extras, and few of us can survive without them. Providing such networks for young isolated mothers and their children in programmes such as Head Start in the USA and Sure Start in the UK includes strategies to prevent depression.

Most of us will experience some periods of depression in our lives and most of us will get over them spontaneously and fairly quickly. Indeed, it is possible to think of depression as a necessary and useful human process—a period when we can work through loss, acknowledge it properly, and move forward. At such times we may need to withdraw a bit into ourselves, and some psychoanalysts consider the ability to be depressed as an essential step towards personal maturity. Certainly people who seem immune to sadness or depression strike us as odd. Psychiatrists have spent years trying to make a clear distinction between 'clinical depression' and 'normal depression' and, frankly, have failed. The difference is more one of degree than genetics or symptom pattern. If it goes on and on, or if the symptoms become unbearable, it needs to be treated; if it gets better on its own after a few weeks, then we see it as a normal variation in mood.

Anxiety

Anxiety is fear spread thin. We've all experienced it and it serves a useful purpose. Some degree of anxiety is essential to keep us alert and help us perform (fear of failure gets us to work for exams). Studies show that, while performance rises with anxiety up to a point, above a certain level performance plummets. Anxiety disorders are probably about as common as depression but fewer people seek help for them. People with 'Generalized Anxiety Disorder' (GAD) are persistently over-anxious. Most of us experience peaks of anxiety quite often, but in anxiety disorders they don't settle. GAD is exhausting and sufferers cannot sleep or concentrate and usually lose weight. Persisting anxiety often leads to depression.

Phobic anxiety disorders are more noticeable. A phobia simply means an exaggerated fear. Most of us have a phobia—so-called 'simple phobias' start in childhood and are constant through life. Animal phobias are typical examples (spiders, mice, snakes). Mine is a height phobia—I cannot climb towers or go near cliff edges.

Most people live with their simple phobias unless they cause serious inconvenience (e.g. a flying phobia in someone whose job requires increased travel, a needle phobia in a woman who becomes pregnant and needs to have blood tests). Simple phobias are remarkably responsive to behaviour therapy using 'graded exposure'. You follow a preset scheme increasing your exposure while monitoring your own anxiety (e.g. start with holding a picture of a spider then hold a small dead one, a larger dead one, a living one in a glass, a living one free, and then a tarantula!).

Most of the phobias seen by psychiatrists are not simple phobias, but either agoraphobia or social phobia. These start in adult life, but fluctuate with stress), and can be quite disabling. Agoraphobia (more often now referred to as a panic disorder) is not fear of open spaces, as many think, but of crowds and crowded places. It comes from the Greek word *Agoros* for market place, not the Latin word *Ager* for field. Agoraphobia predominantly affects women and it is much less common than a generation ago. It is associated with panic attacks and often leads to staying in and avoiding crowds. It is this 'avoidance' that makes the disorder continue. Panic attacks are awful (racing heart, sweating, a dry mouth, and conviction that one is going to faint, wet oneself, or even die). It is no surprise that people escape such situations as fast as possible. The pity is that if they stayed they would soon realize that panic is very short-lived (a matter of minutes, not hours) and fades on its own. However, when we rush off and the panic stops, we become convinced that it was the getting away that stopped it and we don't learn that it was fading anyway. The memory of the last panic starts to get us anxious as we approach the situation again and this 'fear of the fear' increases the likelihood of another attack.

Treatment using behaviour therapy involves teaching the person how to stay with a panic attack and thereby experience its reduction, although it is generally more complicated than with simple phobias. Social phobia is an exaggerated anxiety on meeting new people. There is some real controversy about whether this is a legitimate diagnosis or simply severe shyness, and particularly whether it should be treated with drugs (Chapter 6). In social phobia the problem is usually one of avoidance rather than panic and the treatment includes learning new techniques for approaching social situations.

Obsessive compulsive disorder

Most of us have experienced obsessional behaviour as children—avoiding the cracks in the pavement is the commonest. Sportsmen and actors are notorious for their rituals—the tennis player who *has* to bounce the ball three times before serving, the leading lady who cannot sing without something green in her costume. These superstitious behaviours have much in common with obsessive compulsive disorder (OCD). The patient has to repeat activities or thoughts (most often hand washing or checking and counting rituals) a set number of times or in a set sequence to ward off anxiety. In the obsessional form (where there are often no external rituals) the problem is repetitive thoughts, often about awful outcomes (contamination with dirt or germs, or a fear of shouting out something blasphemous or offensive). The hallmark of OCD is that the thoughts or actions are *repeated*, *resisted*, and *alien* (they appear to be imposed on the patient). They aren't a harmless superstition or quirk, but can dominate and ruin lives. Compulsive cleaners, for instance, end up exhausted because they are never finished cleaning over and over again. Obsessional ruminators cannot hold down a job because they are distracted with repeating their thoughts or counting and they may wear out their partners seeking constant reassurance about their worries.

OCD tends to be associated with specific personality traits—neat, tidy, conscientious people. Most of us recognize obsessional features in ourselves and yet the full disorder seems so bizarre. Indeed, sufferers are often slow to seek help because the symptoms seem so strange and incomprehensible—they are embarrassed by them. OCD has been subject to psychological over-interpretation (Chapter 4) and only recently have effective treatments been developed (behaviour therapy and, in milder cases, antidepressants).

Hysterical disorders

Hysteria is no longer a fashionable term. It has been misused disparagingly to mean over-emotional (and usually of women)—'Oh don't be so hysterical!' Hysterical disorders were originally thought to be restricted to women (*hysteros* is the Greek word for womb). In psychiatry, however, hysteria has played an important role—particularly in psychoanalysis (Chapter 4).

Hysterical disorders are most often striking physical or neurological symptoms for which no organic cause can be found. In 'conversion' disorders anxiety or conflict is expressed as ('converted into') a pain or disability. The most dramatic are paralyses or blindness. The patient insists that they cannot see or move their arm and yet all tests indicate that they 'really' can. In 'dissociative' disorders patients deal with their conflicts by insisting that they are not in touch with some aspect of their mental functioning ('dissociated' from it). In the most extreme case an individual may insist they have multiple personalities and are not responsible for what different 'personalities' do. One of the surprising features of hysterical disorders is that the patient appears relatively content with what looks to others to be a very frightening condition. Charcot, the great 19th-century French neurologist, called this contentment 'la belle indifférence'.

Conversion and dissociation mechanisms are very common (and temporarily often very helpful) in times of enormous stress. Soldiers in war often carry on apparently calm under fire but afterwards have absolutely no memory of it. Most of us have developed a terrible headache or felt unwell inexplicably only later to realize that it was a way of avoiding something we couldn't face. In some cases we may doubt if the mechanism is fully unconscious, as when it is used as a legal defence (e.g. automatism in murder trials).

Hysteria in adults is getting less common in more 'psychologically sophisticated' societies. In the First World War soldiers, unable to acknowledge their terror, developed shell shock (a coarse shaking of the hands and 'jumpiness') which was undoubtedly hysterical. They were genuinely unaware (were 'unconscious') that the fear of battle caused their symptoms. By the Second World War it was widely understood that soldiers could be terrified in battle. Those who could not cope did not develop shell shock but 'combat stress'. They felt the terror and could not function, but they recognized what it was and asked for help. They did not have to deny the fear and convert it into 'acceptable' symptoms such as tremor or paralysis. While conversion symptoms are relatively rare now in psychiatric wards, they are common in general medicine where the less stigmatizing term 'somatization' is used to cover medically unexplained symptoms or those where there is clearly thought to be a significant emotional component. Treatment includes identifying the stresses and helping the patient find other ways of dealing with them or cognitive behaviour therapy and sometimes antidepressants if there is an underlying disorder.

Personality disorders

We all have a personality. Even when we say someone has 'no personality', we mean he has a dull personality. Personality is the collection of characteristics that distinguishes us from each other. It's generally how we first think of people or describe them. Psychiatrists inevitably became interested in personality. First because they have to distinguish between illness and personality (is this person suffering from a depression or are they always morose and pessimistic?). But they also soon noted that there were specific personality types that were associated with the disorders they treated, and for this reason they used the same or similar terms. Thus the schizoid personality is rather distant and strange and the paranoid personality is over-sensitive and prone to suspicion. The hysterical is prone to intense fluctuating emotions, needing passionate relationships and to be the centre of attention, whereas the obsessional is careful and inflexible. The psychopathic personality (variously relabelled sociopathic and antisocial) is not just a delinquent but shows an absence of empathy or remorse. They differ from ordinary criminals such that prisons struggle to deal with them.

The role of psychiatry in the treatment of extremes of personality, 'personality disorders' (PD), is controversial (Chapter 6), and most psychiatrists are sceptical that we have particularly effective treatments. However, personality affects everything about us and so the treatment of any psychiatric disorder will require proper attention to personality. Different societies present problems for different personalities and the classification of personality disorders is changing. The difference between the sexes in the distribution of the two most prominent diagnoses is striking. Currently, women are much more likely to be diagnosed with 'borderline' PD (fluctuating, intense emotions and difficult, dependent relationships, self-harm and low self-esteem, rather similar to the old-term 'hysterical' PD) and men with 'antisocial' PD (violence, delinquency, and impulsiveness quite similar to 'psychopathic' PD). It is not hard to see how these two disorders could be seen as manifestations of the same sense of personal alienation and disappointment but expressed differently because of how our culture moulds the behaviours of men and women.

Addictions

It is far from clear what psychiatry's role should be in the treatment of alcohol and drug abuse. Most people who abuse them do not have mental illnesses. However, there are a number of compelling reasons why psychiatry is involved. People with mental health problems have a very much increased risk of turning to drink or drugs, possibly to dull the pain (particularly in depression and personality disorders). Drug and alcohol abuse also makes recovering from mental illness much more difficult. It is almost impossible to recover fully from depression while drinking to excess, and young schizophrenia patients who abuse drugs find it difficult to cooperate with treatment and attain control of their illnesses.

Addictions can also *cause* mental illnesses. Severe alcohol abuse can lead to paranoid psychoses, delirium tremens, depression, and eventually dementia. Amphetamine and cocaine are associated with quite severe paranoid disorders which can result in violence; acute psychotic reactions are common with LSD and Ecstasy. In addition the poverty and social chaos associated with illegal drug use can lead to depression and despair. So psychiatry is inevitably involved with treating alcohol and drug misuse. However, whether psychiatry should lead it, or simply be one of a range of inputs available to help, can be debated, as can the benefit of classifying addictions as illnesses.

Suicide

Suicide is a tragic, but not infrequent, occurrence in psychiatry. About a quarter of those who commit suicide are in current contact with psychiatrists, and in the UK two-thirds have consulted their GP in the last month (40 per cent in the last week). The psychiatric disorders with the highest immediate risk for suicide are alcoholism and depression, although it is increasingly recognized as a long-term risk in psychotic disorders and anorexia nervosa. Although suicide attempts are more common in young people and women, completed suicides are three times as common in men and overall increase steadily with age. Because of the distress and stigma associated with suicide (attempted suicide has been punished as a crime in many societies and was illegal in the UK up till the 1960s), it has been suggested that almost all suicides result from mental illness.

The French sociologist Durkheim's book *Le Suicide* published in 1897 offered a dramatically different perspective. It focused on the different rates of suicide reported for Catholics and Protestants and emphasized the importance of social isolation. Durkheim believed Catholicism protected from suicide. Catholic countries indeed do report lower suicide rates, but this may reflect a reluctance to admit the cause of death.

There are large variations in suicide rates between different countries and the figures are pretty unreliable. Contrary to an enduring myth, Sweden has never had the highest suicide rate in Europe but rather the countries of central and eastern Europe—e.g. Hungary, Poland, Russia. Not all the differences are just reporting practices. The same national rankings are maintained in immigrants to the USA from these different countries.

It could be argued that suicide is not primarily a psychiatric issue, but psychiatry's intervention has helped reduce rates. There is no specific 'anti-suicide treatment', but the development of anti-suicide policies and improved identification and treatment of mental illnesses have had positive effects. There is no truth in the old wives' tale that those who talk about it don't do it (as the 40 per cent consulting their GP in the preceding month testifies). Teaching GPs on a Swedish island to actively enquire about depression and suicidal thinking and then treat the depression produced a marked fall in the suicide rate.

There are also known risk periods (e.g. just after discharge from psychiatric hospital) when extra support can make a difference. The suicidal impulse is not static—it comes and goes. Consequently, simply making it more difficult does reduce the risk—reducing the pack size of dangerous painkillers has significantly reduced deaths in the UK as has replacing toxic coal-gas with safe North Sea gas. Programmes to block access to deadly pesticides have been successful in limiting the epidemic of suicide in poor, indebted farmers in India. Even netting off bridges helps—introducing delay and time to reflect, allowing the impulse to fade. The worldwide access to help lines such as the Samaritans who offer a sympathetic ear attests to the need to talk things through and make human contact.

While the last century saw an overall decline in the suicide rate (with two marked dips during the wars), there is continuing cause for concern. There has been a steady rise, worldwide, in suicides in young men often attributed to a 'crisis in masculinity' and unemployment. Rates in some high-risk groups (small farmers, young south Asian women) are still alarmingly high. Some of this is due to easy access to lethal means (pesticides and shotguns for farmers and an increasing use of car exhaust fumes), but some is probably due to weakening family ties, a sense of powerlessness, plus widening drug and alcohol misuse.

Perhaps even more significant is the change in society's attitudes towards suicide. While still desperately traumatic for the family, it now attracts little stigma. Indeed it is increasingly seen as just one more option available to individuals with serious and painful illnesses (always a high-risk group) or those who feel their life has run its course. Switzerland and the Benelux countries and some US states have legalized assisted suicide in such cases. Patients with mental illnesses have generally been excluded, but this is no longer so in Holland and Belgium. As living wills become increasingly accepted, and if legally assisted suicide spreads wider (as it undoubtedly will), suicide may be viewed as a moral and ethical issue of personal autonomy rather than a psychiatric problem. In which case it becomes even more important that suicide resulting from mental illness should be prevented where possible to protect such true autonomy.

Why is psychiatry a medical activity?

It is not accepted by everybody (including many within the services themselves) that mental health services should be run by psychiatrists. Are these 'mental health services' or 'psychiatric services'? Much of the controversy focuses on the 'medical model' which is thought to be too narrow and too powerful (Chapter 3). Psychology and social care can both make a strong case to offer the lead, and mental health nursing often stresses its independence. It will be obvious from what has been said so far that good practice requires a broader focus than just medicine. So how did psychiatry become so dominant?

One argument is the overlap between mental and physical diseases. Nearly all mental disease states can be mimicked by physical diseases, and a failure to diagnose these may carry real risks. Thyroid disorders can present as depression or as an anxiety state. Deficiency of the B vitamin Niacin can present as dementia; myasthenia gravis and early multiple sclerosis can easily be misdiagnosed as hysterical disorders. The list is extensive. This is, however, a pretty poor argument. Most patients come to mental health services via their family doctor, who should identify such physical problems. Where this hasn't happened it soon becomes clear that a patient is 'not like the other depressives' and a medical or neurological opinion easily obtained. This may have been a more convincing argument when psychiatric patients were isolated in large mental hospitals but is hardly relevant in the 21st century.

A second argument is that many of the most successful treatments have been developed using a medical approach and, as many of these are drugs, you need a doctor to manage the treatment. The second part of this is not so convincing—psychiatrists attend and prescribe for various facilities such as nursing homes and autism schools without being in charge. However, there is an argument that the 'medical model' has been very successful. By the medical model I mean an approach that, although drawing heavily on scientific theory, is fundamentally pragmatic. If it works, keep doing it; if it doesn't, stop it; if you're not sure, conduct a careful experiment to find out. This commitment to careful collection of evidence and a rigorous structured approach to assessing the strength of that evidence is now well established in medicine. The growth of Evidence Based Medicine (EBM) is one of the 20th century's most successful tools in improving outcomes and removing outmoded and ineffective treatments.

Psychiatry's overall independence from a defining theory, and its broadly scientific approach with a commitment to EBM, are probably its major claims to leadership in this area. There is also within it a benign paternalism and willingness to accept responsibility that, while publicly decried, is often privately welcomed.

A consultation with a psychiatrist

What will happen if your GP refers you to a psychiatrist? Practice varies but follows a broadly predictable pattern. It will almost certainly be an interview—most consultations are entirely conversational with no physical examinations or blood tests. It will usually last between 30 and 60 minutes. It is also likely, as we mentioned before, that the psychiatrist will be a woman. Women now account for over 50 per cent of psychiatrists in most countries with the proportion rising fast. In many modern services a referral to a psychiatrist may go direct to a psychologist or nurse or social worker. But here we will focus on a psychiatric assessment.

The first thing the psychiatrist is likely to do is ask you to tell her in your own words what has been going on, what is distressing you, and what you think the problem is. Although the GP will have summarized this in the referral letter, most of us like to hear it directly from you to get a clear picture. From then on the psychiatrist is likely to steer the discussion to get a broader picture of you and your life (your 'history'). She will find out about your upbringing and your family and usually ask detailed questions about family illnesses (especially psychiatric ones). After that she will ask about your health—both physical and psychiatric—over your lifetime and (particularly in younger people) about drug and alcohol use, as these often have a major impact on psychiatric problems. More detailed questioning is likely about areas relevant to your specific problem (important relationships, work stresses, etc.). Contrary to popular myth you will not be grilled on your sex life!

After taking a history the psychiatrist conducts what is called a 'mental state assessment'. This is a detailed evaluation of your symptoms—worries, mood, sleep, preoccupations. Usually this is also carried out as a conversation although sometimes there may be some quite formal questions and simple tests of memory. These are generally brief and not difficult—it's not like doing an IQ test.

After taking a history and conducting a mental state examination the psychiatrist will usually have come to an opinion of what the problem is (often called a 'formulation'). This formulation usually includes a diagnosis plus much more, such as thoughts about current difficulties and stresses that have brought on the problem. She will discuss these with you to get your opinion and then talk through the various options she thinks possible. This can involve a range of treatments (talking or tablets) or, rarely, a hospital admission. Surprisingly often, advice and reassurance are all that is needed. Nearly a quarter of referrals to psychiatrists in the UK are one-off consultations resulting in advice to the patient or GP.

Because so many psychiatric problems affect family members, psychiatrists will often want to talk with them, both to get a clearer understanding of what is going on but also to explain any proposed treatments to them (they may be very worried) and how best to help. Obviously patients have the right to total confidentiality, but it can be helpful to discuss things more widely.

What the psychiatrist will *not* do is read your mind or ask trick questions. Sometimes it can seem this way because she appears to know much more than you've told her. There is nothing magical about this—it is simply that she will have heard similar stories before and will understand what is going on. That is, after all, her job—to know what depression and anxiety feel like and know how most people cope with such difficulties in their lives. Many find this, in itself, reassuring—that their problems are not unique; others have had similar difficulties and got over them. Psychiatrists have no wish to 'catch you out' with trick questions. They want to know what you are going through and give advice on how to manage it. What will also not happen is a sudden admission to hospital against your will. There are no psychiatric diagnoses that require immediate compulsory hospitalization. That only happens when there is overwhelming evidence of real risk and usually after much discussion with you and with extensive involvement of family and GP.

Having made her assessment and discussed the treatment with you, she may make a further appointment either for you to see her or another member of the team for treatment (e.g. a nurse or psychologist) or alternatively say that you don't need to come back. Whichever happens, she will write to your GP and keep him informed.

So we now know a bit about the scope of psychiatry—how it fits into the other approaches to understanding the mind, what sort of disorders or illnesses it treats, and the major treatment approaches. You may by now regret having started reading—so many uncertainties and contradictions. Couldn't it have been simpler? Well probably not. If we were to invent psychiatry from scratch it might be different. What we have, however, developed organically over the last two centuries. It is the product of powerful competing forces and momentous historical developments and is confronted just now by exciting advances in the neurosciences. So keep reading and by the end it should make some sort of sense—you will remember that you were never promised certainty.

Chapter 2
Asylums and the origins of psychiatry

Psychiatry's history is manageably short—barely 200 years. The mentally deranged have always been recognized and where they could not be cared for within the family some makeshift provision was made—private madhouses and spas for the rich and workhouses for the poor. Workhouses contained everyone who could not care for themselves—the feeble-minded, the sick, the feckless, and the unemployed. Conditions were grim (deliberately so to discourage the burden on the public purse) and the mentally ill often fared badly from other inmates who abused or took advantage of them. Private madhouses were hardly that much better. There was no training required to own or run them. Their main purpose seemed to be to hide mad members of rich families from view, either to protect reputation or to appropriate their fortunes. The harsh treatment of the much-loved King George III generated powerful antipathy towards them in late 18th-century England.

Bedlam was the first major public madhouse. Established in 1247 as a priory and first recorded as housing the mentally ill in 1377, it became a formal public madhouse in 1634. It is still in existence as the much-reformed Bethlem Royal Hospital. The exhibition of the inmates was a popular public pastime in the early 18th century and generated revulsion in educated quarters.

France had established its Hôtel Dieu and Hôpital Général in 651 and 1656 which, despite their names, were not hospitals as we would understand them, but general establishments for custodial care of the destitute, more akin to workhouses. Tollhäuser ('fools' houses') had been established in medieval Europe. The first US insane ward was established in a Boston almshouse in 1729 and the first US psychiatric hospital in 1773 in Williamsburg, Virginia.

The York retreat

The impetus to separate off the mentally ill and provide more appropriate care came not from doctors but from social reformers and reflected an emerging concern with the dignity of man. In our risk-obsessed days it is sobering to realize that asylums were proposed more to protect the deranged individual from society than vice versa. In Paris in 1792, Pinel dramatically and symbolically removed the chains from inmates in the Bicêtre, and in England a Quaker family, the Tukes, built the first recognizable asylum in York. The Tukes were convinced by the writings of Pinel and Esquirol that a calm and harmonious environment, close to nature and with kindness and predictable routines ('moral therapy'), would bring peace to a troubled mind. The York Retreat was built to contain thirty patients. It was opened in 1796 and achieved remarkable results—all the first patients were discharged home improved or even cured. It attracted attention from all over the world and visitors came from the USA and throughout Europe to study and replicate it. The UK developed a liberal regime from the start, reluctant to use mechanical restraints such as chains or belts (later championed by John Conolly in the 'non-restraint movement').

The asylum movement

In the 1820s the asylum movement began in earnest and over the next seventy years hundreds were built (Figure 1). The scale of investment is hard to conceive of now, with enormous,

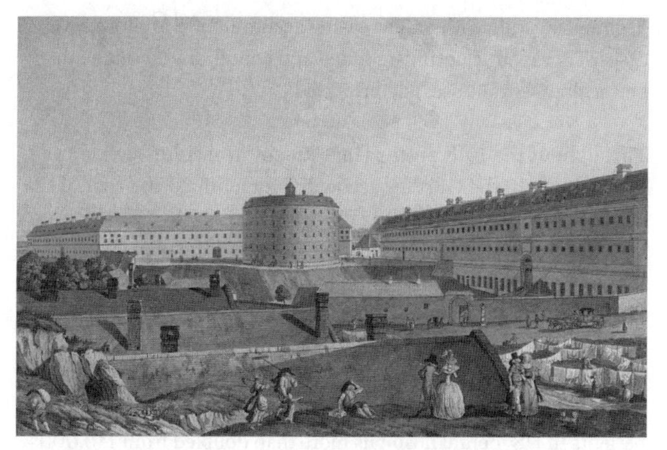

1. Narrenturm ('Fools' Tower') situated alongside the Vienna General Hospital.

well-appointed buildings to house several hundred patients each. The physical conditions within the asylum (space, heating, food, recreation) were significantly better than at home for most patients. The principles of moral therapy dictated that asylums should be spacious, away from busy towns, placed in the countryside with extensive grounds. High, airy locations were selected because of theories current then implicating mists and 'miasmas' in disease.

Doctors were put in charge of asylums primarily because they were easy to hold accountable to a board of governors. There were few effective medical interventions, and the medical superintendent's role was predominantly administrative and disciplinary. He (it was always a 'he') had no power to admit or discharge patients—that was usually held by local magistrates.

Asylums started well, often admitting recent cases—many of whom recovered. They soon seized up, however, filled with those who did not recover. Throughout the latter part of the 19th century and early 20th century, the recovery rate in mental hospitals declined steadily with an increasing accumulation of more severe cases. Therapeutic optimism faded and conditions (though still better than workhouses) deteriorated.

Throughout the 19th century investment in asylums was maintained. In the UK they accounted for a full 20 per cent of county revenues. Their status was promoted in the USA by the influential social reformer Dorothea Dix and the physician Benjamin Rush and in England by the towering social reformer Lord Shaftesbury. Initially quite small institutions, they rapidly grew to several hundred inmates in Europe and up to several thousand in the USA, where the building programme started later and continued longer. Between 1903 and 1933 the number of patients in US mental hospitals more than doubled from 143,000 to 366,000. Most of these were in institutions of more than 1,000 beds, and US mental hospitals continued to expand. The record for the largest was Pilgrim State Hospital in New York which housed over 13,000 patients in 1955 (Figure 2).

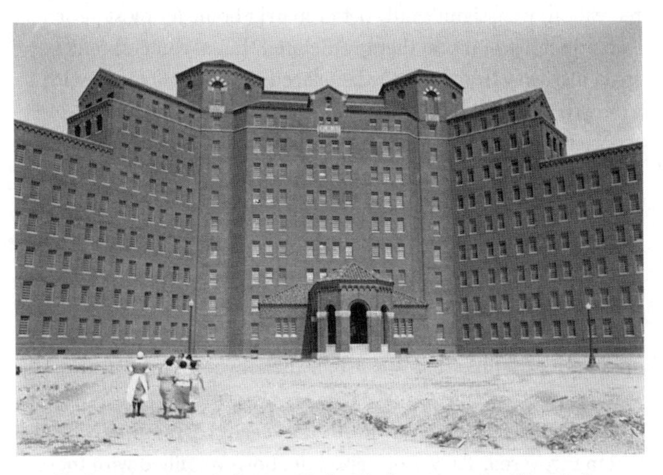

2. Pilgrim State Hospital, New York. The largest mental hospital ever built (13,000 patients in 1955).

The non-restraint movement

Cultural values strongly influence the care of the mentally ill. At the start of the asylum movement the UK and USA focused on human rights and, particularly in the UK, on treating patients with as little physical restriction as possible. John Conolly, the physician superintendent of London's Hanwell Asylum, became the leading proponent of managing patients without straitjackets or chains. He emphasized the value of well-trained and unflappable staff, using isolation to allow patients to calm down. A US visitor commented that the approach would 'never work at home'. This tradition has continued and the UK became the first country to run some mental hospitals entirely without locked doors. Dingleton in Scotland was a fully 'open-door' hospital by 1948—*before* effective drugs (see Chapter 3). The UK approach remains unusual in its total absence of mechanical restraints for agitated patients. Whether its reliance on medication to achieve this is always a good thing is, of course, open to question.

Psychiatry as a profession

Medical superintendents were responsible for running the asylums—ensuring there was enough food, sacking drunken staff, preventing abuse, and proposing discharge to the board when patients recovered. Some of the more able (such as Conolly) became highly skilled in man-management and also took a leading role in the design of new asylums. The early asylum movement produced some remarkable architectural achievements but relatively few therapeutic ones. There was no specific training to be an asylum doctor—you simply worked alongside a superintendent and, if you were lucky, you eventually replaced him. These were, however, generally thoughtful men (they were all men) and interested in science. In the 1840s they founded their own professional bodies across Europe and the USA. The Association of Medical Superintendents in the UK (1841) later became the Royal Medical Psychological Society (1865) and then the Royal College of Psychiatrists (1971).

'Germany'—psychiatry's birthplace

In the second half of the 19th century there was a remarkable intellectual flourishing in German-speaking Europe. The collection of states that came to make up modern Germany were characterized by competing local centres of government with prestigious universities and institutions. Unlike France at the time (where almost everything happened in Paris), there were several independent German-speaking centres of innovation—Munich, Berlin, Vienna, Zurich. From these came the great founding fathers of modern psychiatry: Griesinger, Morel, Alzheimer, Kraepelin, Bleuler, Freud, Jung. The first Germanic professor of psychiatry was appointed in Berlin (Griesinger 1864) with five more by 1882. Compare this to England where the first professor of psychiatry was appointed in 1948.

These academic posts were not, on the whole, placed in mental hospitals nor were they dedicated to the treatment of the legions of psychotic and demented patients who inhabited them. Most research was conducted in university clinics and most was focused on detailed physical examinations of the nervous system in an attempt to elucidate the mechanisms of the 'degeneration' thought to underlie mental illnesses.

Three of psychiatry's most influential figures found their way into the area for more personal reasons. Falling in love was the reason for both Kraepelin and Freud and family concern for Bleuler. Freud and Kraepelin had successful research posts in university departments (Freud was dissecting the nervous system of eels). A research career at that time was incompatible (in terms of both income and time) with family life. However, both had met the women they wanted to marry, so there was no alternative but to look for a 'real job'. Luckily, both had long and happy marriages. Bleuler was born and brought up near Zurich and didn't want to move. His sister suffered from schizophrenia and he took a job at the Burghölzi hospital where she was cared for. These three men moulded modern psychiatry.

Emil Kraepelin (1856–1926)

Kraepelin moved with his new wife in 1886 to become an asylum doctor in Dorpat in what is now Estonia. The professional classes spoke German, but he could not understand his patients' Estonian. What he did do was study their case notes and observe the fluctuations in their illnesses. From this he made the distinction between schizophrenia (which he called 'dementia praecox', meaning early dementia) and manic depressive disorder. Although in their acute phases it was difficult to distinguish the two disorders, important differences emerged over time. The dementia praecox patients rarely or never fully recovered (he believed) and with each bout of acute illness became more disabled. Based on the course of the illnesses he established the classification into the two major functional psychoses that persists to this day.

'Kraeplinian' now implies a pessimistic view of schizophrenia, exaggerating its difference from manic depressive disorder. However, demonstrating that you could classify the psychoses at all was a massive step forward. Distinguishing different patient groups leads to sensible predictions about outcome ('prognosis') and a clearer picture of each illness. It prompted psychiatrists to start distinguishing the others (dementia, cerebral syphilis, intoxications). Diagnosis gave psychiatry a reason to pay more attention to patients' illnesses, rather than just warehousing them, and provided a basis for some rudimentary predictions and the development of treatments. Kraepelin's influential textbook was reprinted for decades.

Eugen Bleuler (1857–1939)

Bleuler first coined the term schizophrenia in 1911. It followed many years of careful study in the Burghölzi hospital in Zurich. Bleuler's situation could hardly have been more different from Kraepelin's. He had grown up using the same Swiss dialect as his patients, lived in the hospital where his sister was a patient with schizophrenia, and often spent evenings talking to his patients. He wanted to understand, to make sense of, his patients' inner world rather than just observe like Kraepelin. His definition of schizophrenia is based on the patient's experience. This approach allowed him to make the diagnosis even if the outcome was good. Of course there remained many schizophrenia patients with poor outcomes, but Bleuler confirmed that some did recover.

Bleuler considered that the primary disturbances in schizophrenia were a withdrawal from close relationships and disturbances of thinking and mood. He believed that hallucinations and delusions were attempts by the patient to make sense of these primary experiences. His definition rested on 'Four As'. These are *Autism* (withdrawal), *Affect* (mood disturbances), *Association* (thought disorder—different associations or meanings being attached to words), and *Ambivalence* (lack of direction and motivation). Bleuler's approach has been superseded in recent years by a focus on the 'positive' symptoms (delusions, hallucinations, thought disorder) because of their greater ease of recognition and responsiveness to drug treatment. His was certainly a more humane approach to this, the most devastating of the mental illnesses. He accorded meaning to the experiences of even his most deteriorated patients.

Sigmund Freud (1856–1939)

Like Kraepelin, Freud had to abandon his preferred career for marriage, pursuing the only option for a Jewish doctor in Vienna at that time, namely private practice. Freud had little experience of asylums and worked almost exclusively with neuroses. He always recognized the limitations of his approaches for more severely ill patients. However, a careful reading of his case histories leaves little doubt that he treated some pretty disturbed individuals. His investigations took him in a completely different direction: the founding of psychoanalysis (Chapter 3). He thought of himself as much as a scientist exploring the mind as a doctor curing illnesses. He always believed that physical treatments (medicines) would eventually be the remedy.

We might anticipate antagonism between these groups a century ago but this doesn't appear so. This was a pre-drug psychiatry. All that was available to doctors after they had classified their patients into broad diagnostic groups was to talk with them. Moral therapy evolved into a rough and ready psychotherapy. Few believed this cured the disease, but the role of doctors has never been restricted to just cure, but also to bringing relief from suffering. The journals of asylum doctors of this period record the time spent talking with patients—attempting to bring comfort and using reasoning to calm them.

The work of another great German psychiatrist, Karl Jaspers (1883–1969), exemplifies this. Jaspers wrote his masterpiece in Heidelberg by the age of 30—*General Psychopathology* (1913). This book has never been out of print nor ever bettered as a description of the mental processes in psychotic illnesses. Jaspers was initially quite comfortable with the writings of psychoanalysts and he recognized two different approaches to researching mental illnesses. The first is *verstehen* 'understanding' and the second *erklären* 'explaining'. He considered both legitimate and necessary, 'what is the meaning of what the patient says and what is causing it?' This dichotomy, however, still underlies disputes in psychiatry—particularly between the psychologically minded and the biologically minded. Jaspers eventually lost patience with Freud, who he believed thought that to understand was sufficient to explain. Early psychiatry valued both approaches.

The first medical model

The end of the asylum era (Chapter 3) was foreshadowed by the 'first medical model' in the 1920s and 1930s. Interest in psychiatry had received a boost during the First World War from the need to treat shell-shocked soldiers. Three revolutionary treatments were introduced—malaria treatment for cerebral syphilis in the 1920s and electro-convulsive therapy and insulin coma therapy in the 1930s. These caused widespread changes in attitudes and restored optimism. 'Lunatic' was replaced with 'mental patient', 'asylum' with 'mental hospital', 'certification' with 'involuntary admission'. Voluntary admissions became common for the first time. This was a massive change in mindset.

Julius Wagner-Jauregg (1857–1940) and malaria treatment

Wagner-Jauregg was the first psychiatrist to be awarded the Nobel Prize for Medicine. He received it for his 1917 introduction of malaria treatment for cerebral syphilis (then called general paralysis of the insane, GPI). Before effective treatments for syphilis, the disease affected the brain with disastrous consequences in a small proportion of patients. This often took twenty years to develop, by which time the patient might be a settled family man. At the turn of the century GPI patients constituted over 10 per cent of male asylum admissions and up to 30 per cent in private asylums. The terror it represented for 19th-century society is vividly captured in Ibsen's play *Ghosts*. Onset of mental symptoms was sudden and dramatic. The philosopher Nietzsche inexplicably embraced a horse in the street in Turin and within days was confined to a mental hospital where he died eleven years later. Deterioration was tragic and humiliating. It was often associated with delusions of grandeur (hence the old cartoons of patients convinced they were Napoleon), and ended in dementia.

Wagner-Jauregg's treatment consisted of infecting the patient with malaria parasites with careful nursing through the high fevers. Repeated fevers killed the syphilis germs and the malaria could afterwards be treated with quinine. This treatment was difficult and risky, but the alternative held no hope. GPI was effectively cleared from mental hospitals long before effective antibiotics arrived. Malaria treatment restored optimism and strengthened the professional pride of the doctors and nurses who had to manage this difficult, but effective, treatment. Patients also often had to be treated in general hospitals and it became clear that despite certification they would often cooperate, forcing a rethink about compulsion.

Electro-convulsive therapy

While malaria treatment and insulin coma therapy (see Chapter 6) are purely of historical interest, electro-convulsive therapy (ECT) is still widely used. Psychiatrists knew that epileptic seizures often caused profound changes in mood. It was also believed (incorrectly) that epilepsy was uncommon in patients with schizophrenia, hence the idea that seizures might be protective. Fits were induced in schizophrenia patients from 1935 by getting them to inhale camphor or by injecting a chemical called metrazol. The results were promising, with many patients showing improvement. However, the experience was awful leading up to the fit, with mounting dread after the metrazol injection, so many patients refused treatment.

An Italian, Ugo Cerletti, came up with the idea of using a weak electric current to initiate the fit and used it on his first patient in 1938 with striking results. Several psychiatrists started to use ECT and its results were truly remarkable. It did calm very agitated schizophrenic patients, but its most dramatic results were with depressed patients, many of whom made sustained recoveries. If this all sounds a bit barbaric to us now, it pays to remember that depressed patients in the 1930s (even in very good mental hospitals) often stayed for years and up to one-fifth *died* during the admission.

Initially ECT was given without anaesthetic and clearly was a frightening experience often with complications of headache, memory loss, and even small fractures if the fit was very strong. For the last fifty years patients have received a short-acting anaesthetic and a chemical to block the muscle contractions so there is no fit to see and no risk of fractures. Headache and some memory loss remain concerns, but patients don't recall the actual seizure.

The discovery and durability of ECT is typical of many developments in psychiatry. The idea that started it (that epilepsy protected against schizophrenia) was wrong, but the treatment worked, and in addition it worked better for a different disorder! We still don't know why it works, but it certainly does. It remains one of the most effective treatments in psychiatry and (despite its baleful reputation) the one that most patients who have had it say they would want again.

Mental health legislation

Psychiatry is unique within medicine in being able to compel treatment against a patient's clearly expressed wishes. Consequently most countries have passed specific legislation to permit and monitor it. The whole of the asylum movement was firmly based in such legislation.

The first legislation was to regulate madhouses. All this did was to register them. It set no standards but could close an individual madhouse in the event of flagrant abuse. The purpose of the Asylum Act of 1808 and the Lunacy Act of 1845 was to ensure that care was provided and prevent abuse of the vulnerable mentally ill. It allowed for 'the removal of the furiously mad' to the asylum.

Over the next half century, public concerns shifted from the neglect and abuse of the indigent mentally ill to the spectre of malevolent incarceration of the sane to rob them of their wealth. The 'Alleged Lunatics' Friends Society' (with an admiral of the fleet as chairman) gained considerable parliamentary and public support in late 19th-century Britain. Georgina Weldon (a 'spirited, attractive, wealthy and well connected woman') filled Covent Garden Opera House with an 1883 rally to challenge her recent incarcerations, and eventually won her case. Increasing public disquiet culminated in the 1890 Lunacy Act. This highly legalistic document, several hundred pages and 342 sections long, prioritized the protection of patients' rights to such an extent that early and voluntary treatment became virtually impossible.

So swings the pendulum of public attitudes to mental health. Virtually every developed nation is struggling to balance legal rights and therapeutic needs, to balance society's needs with the patient's. We will return to this in Chapter 6 but it is sobering to be reminded that we have been here before.

Asylums limped on for another 50–60 years, mired in legislation and inhibited from innovation apart from the welcome treatment advances in the 1920s and 1930s. It was to be another thirty years before this awesome international movement was finally challenged and moved towards its end. This is the subject of Chapter 3.

Chapter 3
The move into the community

After decades of being hidden from view, the mentally ill are now very much in the public eye. Hardly a week goes by without some headline about the plight of the homeless mentally ill or an incident involving a disturbed or vulnerable individual (Figure 3). 'Care in the Community' has become an international preoccupation with

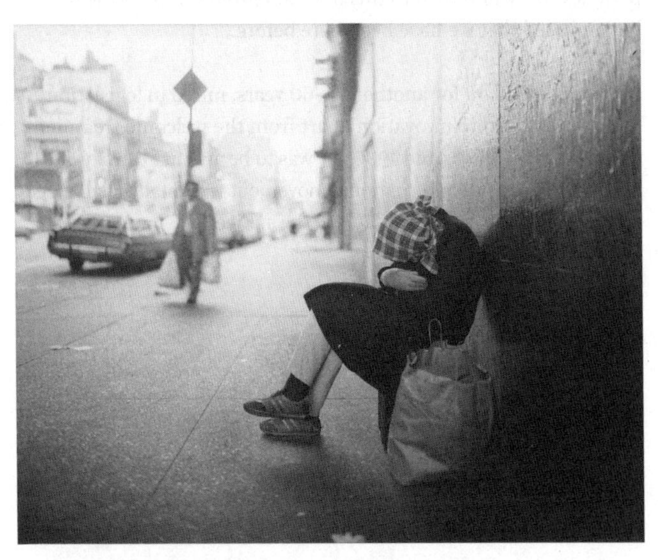

3. A 'bag lady': a homeless, mentally ill woman with her few possessions.

much soul-searching and fear of violence and disorder. How has this situation come about? Is it really so disastrous and, if so, what can be done about it?

Deinstitutionalization

The number of psychiatric beds in the West has shrunk to less than a third of what it was in 1955. Nearly every large mental hospital in the UK and most in the USA and Western Europe have closed. The few remaining house only a fraction of the patients they once did. Chronic wards where long-stay patients lived out impoverished lives have virtually disappeared. In the mid-1950s there were 500,000 psychiatric inpatients in the USA and 160,000 in the UK. Now there are less than 100,000 in the USA and less than 30,000 in the UK. If you adjust for population growth this represents a 90 per cent reduction. This trend is virtually worldwide. This process, inelegantly entitled 'deinstitutionalization', started by reducing overcrowding and then closing wards. The last twenty years has finally seen the closure of whole hospitals.

It is usual to attribute this emptying of the asylums to the discovery of antipsychotic drugs in the early 1950s. This was clearly a major factor, but it is far from the whole story. Fundamental changes in social attitudes towards the mentally ill were afoot before the drugs were introduced. The impact of the new drugs also varied enormously—from wholesale discharges in some countries, to almost no effect in others. Social attitudes and radical rethinking within psychiatry also exerted powerful influences. Later, financial considerations entered the picture. But let us start with the drugs.

The drug revolution

Like so many important discoveries chlorpromazine's antipsychotic effect was found by pure chance. A French navy anaesthetist treating trauma patients noted how it reduced the need for anaesthetic and calmed patients post-operatively without sedating them. Two psychiatrists, Delay and Deneke, tried the drug in St Anne's hospital in Paris in 1952 and were astounded by the results. By the tenth patient they knew they had a breakthrough. Over the next four years chlorpromazine became the front-line treatment in psychotic illnesses. It 'swept like a whirlwind throughout psychiatry' and the atmosphere in wards was totally transformed.

At its most basic the drug humanized care. Staff could begin to get to know their calmer and less distressed patients rather than just controlling them. Episodes of illness were both shorter and less disturbed, so that rehabilitation and early discharge became realistic possibilities before family relationships and jobs were lost for good. Initially, the drugs were used only to treat acute episodes, but by the 1970s it was realized that continuing with them substantially reduced further breakdowns. This 'maintenance therapy' has become the cornerstone of long-term treatment of schizophrenia and other psychoses.

Over the last fifty years a whole range of antipsychotics has been developed. Most are equally effective, but their side effects vary. The original chlorpromazine-like drugs often made patients stiff and lethargic. Newer drugs avoid the stiffness but can cause weight gain and diabetes. Antipsychotics are now available as long-acting injections, which means patients can forget about them other than an injection every two to four weeks.

The drug revolution was not restricted to antipsychotics. The first of the antidepressants (imipramine) was introduced in 1958. These had a longer lasting effect than ECT and were more acceptable to patients. Antidepressant use has increased by 65 per cent in the USA between 1999 and 2014 with one in eight adults reporting recent use. Lithium carbonate (a naturally occurring substance) was noted in 1949 to have a calming effect.

It was introduced as a long-term 'mood-stabilizing' treatment for manic-depressive disorder in 1968 and has substantially reduced the rate of breakdowns.

This is not the place to detail the developments in modern psychiatric drugs but just to note that the progress has been accelerating. We now have a wide range of drugs for most recognized disorders. However, they are not 'magic bullets'. No drug will completely cure all patients with a specific disorder, but, carefully chosen, drug treatments can make a real difference to the vast majority of patients with mental illnesses. The very success of these newer drugs poses significant risks for overuse (Chapter 6).

The revolution in social attitudes

Psychiatry changed radically during the Second World War and gained new confidence from the treatment of combat disorders. Its raised profile brought many doctors into it who would never have contemplated working in asylums. Fresh minds were brought to old problems. Previously healthy men transformed into nervous wrecks by battle challenged older, fatalistic genetic explanations of mental illness. Dramatic successes with practical treatments (e.g. barbiturate injections to release or 'abreact' emotions from recent terrifying experiences) confirmed the role of stress and trauma. Psychiatry became an active and optimistic, even quite glamorous, branch of medicine.

Therapeutic communities

The treatment of acute war neuroses was not the only consequence of the Second World War. Psychiatrists with a psychoanalytical training obtained influential posts as military advisers in both the USA and UK and explored how organizations themselves influenced mental health and recovery. One result was the 'therapeutic community'.

The therapeutic community approach recognizes that the *organization* of hospitals (or prisons or schools or offices for that matter) has a major impact on the well-being of those in them. For psychiatric patients it can be an opportunity for self-learning and recovery. Army psychiatrists found that rank and status got in the way when treating enlisted men. So they minimized status differences, encouraging informality and stressing their patients' capacities to work together and help each other. This allowed demoralized individuals to learn new ways of dealing with their problems in a democratic, optimistic, and enquiring group environment.

The therapeutic community movement improved care in mental hospitals, reducing chronicity and institutionalization. It has become a victim of its own success, as its lessons are so accepted (even in commercial organizations) that their origins are forgotten. Psychoanalysis has suffered a similar fate.

'Institutional neurosis' and 'total institutions'

That traditional mental hospital environments could have a profoundly damaging impact on patients began to be realized in the late 1950s. Hospitals could themselves be the *cause* of some of the problems that they were striving to treat. Long-stay patients (usually with schizophrenia) were commonly apathetic, self-neglecting, and isolated. This had always been considered a consequence of the illness (the 'schizophrenia defect state') and caring for such individuals a further justification of the need for mental hospitals.

Unlike the acute symptoms of hallucinations, delusions, and agitation, this withdrawal responded poorly to the new drugs. However, the hospital environment seemed to make a difference. It had always been known that there were good mental hospitals and bad ones. A study comparing three hospitals in the 1960s found markedly different levels of apathy and self-neglect related to the levels of activity and variety provided in daily routines.

A psychiatrist, Russell Barton, proposed that this was a response to living in institutions which removed personal responsibility. You stopped looking after yourself because somebody else always did it for you. Barton called this 'institutional neurosis' to stress that its cause was the hospital, not the schizophrenia. When he gave his patients more independence many flourished and were soon discharged. With active rehabilitation (helping patients regain their lost skills and abilities) optimism grew that these apathetic, disabled patients would no longer need inpatient care.

The extent of institutional neurosis was undoubtedly exaggerated. There *is* a demotivated state that develops as an integral feature of long-term schizophrenia, but it was undoubtedly magnified by stultifying hospital routines. Some patients had even recovered and the overworked staff had simply not noticed! Many patients embraced their independence effortlessly, but 'overlooked' patients are now rare and most need ongoing support after discharge.

Erving Goffman and total institutions

The Three Hospitals Study and Russell Barton's institutional neurosis book shook up psychiatry but nothing like the international shock wave caused by *Asylums* (1961) by the American sociologist Erving Goffman. This was based on a year working 'undercover' for his PhD in an enormous mental hospital in Washington, DC. His clear and radical conclusions expressed in powerful writing simply stunned the establishment. Goffman described in convincing detail what *really* went on in an asylum—not what people *thought* went on, or what they *meant* to go on. Doctors and nurses thought they shared a common understanding, but Goffman showed that doctors used a disease and treatment model, whereas nurses judged more on patient behaviours and motives. More tellingly, doctors thought they ran the units, but it was clear that for day-to-day life nurses and aides (and even some patients) established the rules and culture and held the authority. Goffman was not sympathetic to the asylum.

He went further. He concluded that the dehumanizing and degradation of patients resulting from inflexible routines were not simply regrettable consequences of poorly trained staff or lack of resources (Russell Barton's explanation). He proposed that they existed to *deliberately* erode individuality. This process was characteristic of what he called 'total institutions' such as asylums, prisons, and the army. These are wrap-round organizations with rigid distinctions between staff and patients (or prisoners and warders, or army officers and men) and demeaning rituals which suppress individual identity. Goffman believed they do this to establish discipline ('break you down to build you up') and thereby make everything more easily manageable. He particularly deplored the highly structured admission process that included not only medical examination but delousing, bathing, and hair cutting for all patients as a potent symbolic degradation.

Whilst (understandably) initially unwelcome to psychiatry, Goffman's writings have been a major force in driving the closure of the mental hospitals. *Asylums* is still *the* most quoted text in modern sociology fifty years after its publication. Ken Kesey's 1962 book *One Flew Over the Cuckoo's Nest* (and its enormously successful film adaptation staring Jack Nicholson in 1975) vividly portrayed the unacceptable face of such large impersonal asylums (Figure 4).

The rights and abuse of the mentally ill

I have focused so far on psychiatry's contribution to deinstitutionalization. However, as with the origins of the asylums (Chapter 2), the social climate was at least as influential, if not

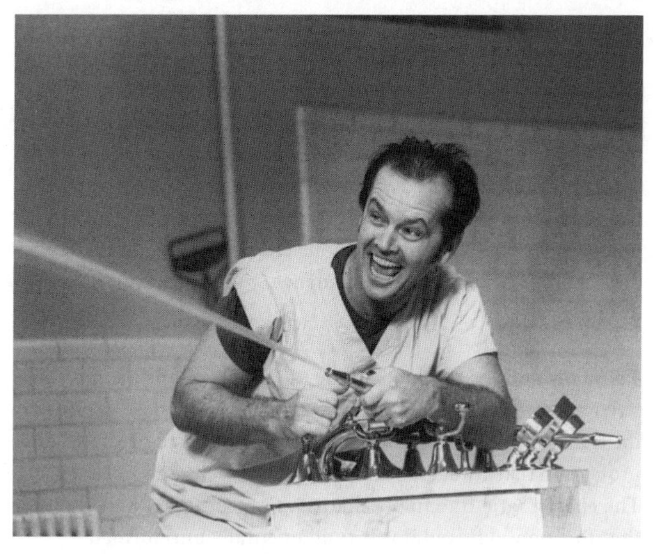

4. ***One Flew Over the Cuckoo's Nest.***

more so. Directly after the Second World War Europe burned with a spirit of change and a thirst for social justice. The old order was in disgrace and the rights of the common man were the priority of both returning soldiers and returned governments. Democracy and social inclusion (though not called that then) dominated the international agenda, whether in education, health, or housing. The rights of disadvantaged groups to take full part in this new society were strongly defended and the mentally ill were one such group. The wholesale liquidation of chronic patients in Nazi Germany only served to underline their need for protection. Nowhere is this new thinking so clearly demonstrated as in changes in Mental Health Law. In the UK, for example, the 1890 Lunacy Act focused on protecting the rights of the sane not to be judged insane (with scant regard to the rights or welfare of the insane), whereas the 1959 Mental Health Act focused on protecting the rights of the mentally ill by ensuring due process and regular reviews of their care and detention.

A series of scandals exposing the abuse of mental patients surfaced soon after the war. Revelation after revelation of degrading and inadequate care prompted several inquiries. The reported abuses ranged from neglect and denial of dignity through to frank mistreatment and assault. These scandals painted a recurrent picture of large, isolated institutions, with a poorly trained but very cohesive staff group, many of whom had followed their parents into the job. The practices Goffman described were very much in evidence, with little attention to humane care.

These revelations produced understandable revulsion and strengthened the resolve to reform or remove asylums. In 1960 the UK Health Minister prophesied their demise but predicted that professional attitudes would outlive the bricks and mortar. The charismatic Italian psychiatrist Franco Basaglia believed that the mental hospital was fundamentally unreformable (see Chapter 5) and abolition was the only way. An Italian law passed in 1978 prohibited compulsory admissions to mental hospitals immediately and required their total closure within three years.

At this time the very legitimacy of psychiatry was being called into question. The anti-psychiatry movement (Chapter 5) spearheaded by R. D. Laing, Thomas Szasz, and Michel Foucault was celebrated in the 1968 student revolts.

By the early 1980s the downsizing and closing of mental hospitals was an established international movement led and articulated mainly by psychiatrists. The cost of mental health care *increased* as staffing standards improved and decades of neglect were addressed. The financial advantages of closing whole mental hospitals became obvious to governments who have now set the agenda over the last thirty years. One astute US observer noted this 'unholy alliance between therapeutic liberals and fiscal conservatives' behind deinstitutionalization.

'Transinstitutionalization' and 'reinstitutionalization'

When the asylums were built they did not take most patients from family homes but from prisons and workhouses. A worrying aspect of deinstitutionalization is that more mentally ill patients end up in prisons. As psychiatric units became smaller and more therapeutic in orientation, more difficult patients (who previously might have remained on locked wards) ended up in prison. This is accelerated where compulsory care requires evidence of immediate danger. California now has more actively psychotic individuals in prison than in mental hospitals.

So deinstitutionalization is not quite so straightforward. Indeed, the last decade has witnessed a slight reverse, with more patients in some form of supervised accommodation. The reasons are complex but one is undoubtedly an increasing intolerance of risk.

Care in the community

'Any fool can close a mental hospital,' remarked a senior UK health official in the 1980s, quickly adding that the real challenge was providing alternative care. Recognizable forms of modern community care have been developing since the 1930s—day hospitals in Russia, outpatient departments in both the USA and the UK, mobile clinics in the Netherlands. However the 1960s onwards sees a step-change in developing community services as an *alternative* to mental hospitals rather than an *addition*.

District general hospital units and day hospitals

The building of small inpatient units either in or alongside local general hospitals was the proposed model to replace the mental hospital and destigmatize mental illness. With 40–100 beds they catered for acute, short-term patients but could rely on mental hospital back-up. Their character varied. In the USA they embodied a long tradition of general hospital liaison psychiatry; in Germany an academic psychosomatic approach including psychotherapeutic treatment of physical illnesses; in the UK a mental hospital tradition adapted to shorter stays. The Italian reforms insisted on a complete break, substituting tiny fifteen-bed units focusing on short-term crisis.

There was, however, no wholesale international replacement of mental hospitals. In Europe over half of psychiatric inpatients are still in traditional mental hospitals with little, if any, real community provision. US practice varies enormously between states, from highly community-based services to extensive reliance on old mental hospitals. Small general hospital units guard against many of the problems of asylums, but bring others, such as being cramped and less tolerant of very difficult patients. They can rarely offer a range of activities and treatments but still represent a first essential step out from the asylum into the community.

Community mental health teams (CMHTs)

New services needed to be more local and acceptable to patients and families. 'Sector psychiatry' arose to meet the challenge. Asylums often took all the patients from a whole county or city. The sector approach divided this into small manageable areas (40,000–100,000 population) with dedicated teams to provide accessible personalized care.

France and the UK led the way in this development. The French 'secteur' was based on sophisticated sociological theory, emphasized crisis intervention restricted to psychotic patients, and was never fully implemented. The UK approach was based on a recognition of the central importance of social care and support systems for reintegrating the mentally ill. It was more comprehensive and pragmatic. Localized care became a practical necessity as 1950s legislation demanded that discharged patients be offered outpatient follow-up by those who discharged them with close involvement of social services. Collaboration was not feasible from distant mental hospitals. Joint working with social workers and family doctors was only manageable across small neighbourhoods. The sector approach meant psychiatrists, nurses, and social workers started working together in teams.

In the UK the engine of this development was the 'community psychiatric nurse' (CPN). CPNs work almost exclusively outside hospital, visiting patients in their homes to provide emotional and practical support and supervision of medication. From just two CPNs in 1953 they now vastly outnumber psychiatrists in the UK and form the backbone of multidisciplinary teams. These teams now include social workers, clinical psychologists, and occupational therapists.

CMHTs assess the whole range of mental health problems (from depression to psychosis) and offer treatment in clinics, patients' homes, day hospitals, and (when needed) as inpatients. They have become the norm throughout Europe and many parts of the world. The Italian reforms most clearly encapsulated this model of care, emphasizing informality, local knowledge, and flexible access.

Most CMHTs are broadly similar. In Italy and in the UK, until recently, the same team looks after patients both in and out of the hospital, but in much of Europe and the USA these responsibilities are separate. Some CMHTs accept the whole range of mental health problems; others restrict themselves to severe psychoses. CMHTs have increasingly separated into a range of specialized teams (e.g. for crisis, for long-term support, for first-onset patients). While the focus of these teams differs, their practices (staffing, assessment, reviews, etc.) are broadly similar.

CMHTs are not the only model for provision of local services. Community Mental Health Centres are larger units providing a range of services including day care, assessment, treatment, and outreach. This model functions well in some parts of Europe and the USA.

Day hospitals

Day hospitals were proposed alongside general hospital units as the early alternative to mental hospitals but have been overtaken somewhat by the rapid development of the CMHT. Many patients with depression and anxiety are now treated by CMHT staff with their expanded skills, and effective outreach to psychosis patients has reduced the need for day hospitals. However day *centres* which provide social rather than health care continue to flourish. They reduce the isolation and loneliness experienced by many mentally ill people, particularly in large anonymous cities.

Stigma and social integration

The first twenty years of the move to community care is generally considered very successful. Patients escaped dismal mental hospitals to more rewarding lives. CMHTs offered effective but light-touch support. As whole mental hospitals eventually began to close, however, patients with increasingly severe disabilities were discharged. Adequate alternative services lagged behind, in particular affordable local housing. Some patients became homeless (particularly in the USA where it became a national scandal). Living in squalor on the streets, often victims of petty crime and exploitation, they stand as a reproach to civilized values. The picture is, of course, very varied, but major cities (London, Rome, New York, Los Angeles) have struggled to cope and generally not succeeded.

Civil liberties legislation, which prevents hospitalization unless there is evidence of immediate danger (as in New York and California), has worsened this problem. Even when there is a bed, these new laws often prevent much needed compulsory admission.

However, it is sobering to reflect that patients often prefer living in poverty and insecurity on the street to a relatively comfortable hospital ward. This cannot simply be written off as lack of insight—most of us value personal freedom and choice above comfort. However, the sight of 'bag-ladies' and homeless, obviously mentally disturbed individuals on our streets presents a sharp moral challenge to which we have no easy answer.

Stigma

Stigma is one of the main burdens of mental illness and there are now international programmes to reduce it. Stigma is manifest by our wish to avoid contact with individuals ('establish social distance') and in its most extreme form to expel or banish them. Mental illness has always been stigmatized, as have many other illnesses in the past. Discrimination and neglect, especially in jobs and housing, still leave the mentally ill denied full social acceptance. Younger people appear to be less rejecting towards the mentally ill. Hopefully, they understand mental illness better, having been more exposed to it in this era of care in the community, although it may be that people simply become more intolerant with age.

We usually try to avoid (i.e. discriminate against or stigmatize) people who we think pose a risk to us. In the past the fear was mainly of infection (leprosy, tuberculosis, etc.), but with mental illness it is of frightening or dangerous behaviour. For most patients any risk is to themselves from suicide or self-harm. Psychosis is, however, associated with a fourfold risk of violent behaviour. While this may seem a lot it is nothing compared to the risk associated with otherwise healthy but intoxicated young men. Rare but shocking cases of homicide by the mentally ill fuel an exaggerated perception of risk leading to restrictive legislation. In the UK wholesale reform of the mental health services was driven by two infamous homicides, one by a neglected individual with schizophrenia and one by a chaotic drug-abusing man.

While each of these individual incidents is a tragedy for all involved, they really do not amount to an epidemic. In England, for example, homicide by the mentally ill has remained constant at about 160 a year for the last fifty years, while homicide by the non-mentally ill has increased from just over 300 a year in 1980 to nearly 800 in 2015. Most of these 'mental illness' homicides occur within the family or are by individuals with personality disorders or drug and alcohol misuse (not what most of us typically think of as 'mental illness'). However, the fear of random assault by a psychotic individual, 'prematurely discharged from a mental hospital', is remarkably potent. In the UK you are more likely to be killed by a speeding police car than by a mentally ill stranger.

Social consensus and the post-modern society

Extreme individualization and risk avoidance are characteristics of our 'post-modern' society. As shared values recede, individual well-being becomes the dominant preoccupation. Whether this argument is convincing or not it is undeniable that Western societies, with massively increased social mobility, are increasingly individualistic and risk-conscious.

Modern industrial societies are rarely 'homogeneous'—there are large sections of society with quite differing origins, religions, values, and ethnicity. Despite its obvious social benefits, such diversity can make psychiatry very difficult. Differing lifestyles and behaviours are accepted as personal choices; tolerated as long as they do not infringe the next person's liberties. Most of us value these freedoms very highly, but they can reduce our recognition of mental illness. It becomes less obvious when strange dress and behaviour signal an illness rather than self-expression. The over-active, disinhibited manic patient may now be simply dismissed as irresponsible or exhibitionist.

Such uncertainty is complicated by a vast increase in alcohol and recreational drug use. Intoxication usually makes mental illnesses worse and their treatment more difficult. It also can delay their recognition. It is depressingly common to assess a young student who has been unwell for months but whose room-mates assumed it was just drug use.

Stigma, an exaggerated sense of risk from the mentally ill, family break-up, high social mobility, and increasing levels of drug and alcohol use all combine to make community care of the mentally ill much more difficult than it was when the process started half a century ago. This is signalled by the small but widespread rise in compulsory treatment and a modest increase in 'reinstitutionalization'. However this is balanced by a much more sophisticated and embedded respect for individual rights than would have been conceivable a generation ago. We can anticipate continued soul-searching about community care and the optimal level of institutional provision. However any large-scale return to long-stay institutions is unlikely. Community care in one form or another is with us for the foreseeable future.

Chapter 4

Psychoanalysis and psychotherapy

Psychotherapy means different things to different people. Literally it means 'treatment of the mind', though it can be read as 'treatment *by* the mind'. I will use this second understanding (otherwise all psychiatric activity would be psychotherapy and we would be no further forward). In this chapter psychotherapy will include any deliberate, structured use of the *relationship* between a therapist and patient to promote change or better self-understanding. Psychotherapy is usually conducted by talking, hence the current expression 'talking treatments', but in some therapies words are not the crucial element and in some the 'dialogue' is internal. The psychotherapies are dealt with in greater detail in *Psychotherapy: A Very Short Introduction.*

How is psychotherapy different from normal kindness?

Much of what characterizes psychotherapy characterizes normal life. We all try to help our friends and family by being supportive and talking things through when they are upset. Asylum doctors used to spend considerable time in with their patients to calm and reassure them. This was broadly psychotherapeutic in aim. What is special about psychotherapies, however, is that there is an explicit *agreement*, almost a contract, between patient and therapist to *concentrate* on it and set aside specific times for it. Each psychotherapy also follows a recognized and agreed approach, with some understanding about what will happen and how long it will take.

Terms such as 'talking treatments' or 'psychological treatments' are used to avoid old sectarian arguments about what is 'true' psychotherapy. The NHS has a rather helpful hierarchy:

Type A comprises simple psychotherapeutic understanding employed during any treatment (e.g. counselling and support from a doctor prescribing antidepressants).

Type B involves dedicated sessions devoted exclusively to psychological understanding and emotional support. These use general psychotherapeutic principles but don't adhere to a strict theory or have a prescribed number of sessions. An example would be a nurse having regular meetings with a depressed patient on the ward to talk through her sense of loss.

Type C treatments are 'psychotherapy proper'. Here the therapist has a recognized psychotherapy training and there is a clear, shared undertaking to pursue a specified course of that psychotherapy.

Some of the practices common in earlier (psychodynamic) psychotherapies are used in Type A and Type B treatments and usually go unrecognized unless applied in 'proper' Type C psychotherapies.

Sigmund Freud and the origins of psychoanalysis

No story of psychotherapy can ignore Sigmund Freud. Love him or loathe him, he is a towering figure who has radically altered not just psychotherapy but much of how the Western world thinks. We met him in Chapter 2, forced to leave his research and make a living for himself in private practice in Vienna. Most of his clientele were 'neurotic' and most were female. The commonest problems he saw were either 'neurasthaenia' (lack of motivation, mild to moderate depression) or a series of ostensibly physical complaints (paralyses, pains, seizures, etc.) for which there was no identifiable physical cause. Before reaching Freud these patients would have been subject to exhaustive medical examinations and exotic treatments without benefit.

In over fifty years' practice and twenty-four volumes of writing, Freud's ideas changed significantly and they are sometimes contradictory. The outline that follows is, of necessity, simplified and partial but there are many detailed and accessible introductions (e.g. Anthony Storr's *Freud: A Very Short Introduction*).

Freud was heavily influenced by the scientific thinking of his time. Darwin's *Origin of Species* had located mankind squarely in the natural world (no longer a unique divine creation) so the mind became a legitimate subject for scientific investigation. The laws of thermodynamics (that energy is never lost—simply transformed) underpinned 19th-century Europe's economic expansion. Whether water, steam, or internal combustion engines, these new machines drew upon damming up energy and channelling its release. Freud's ideas of the human mind are shot through with this metaphor of blocked instinctual drives or repressed memories. He believed mankind's destructive and creative capacities stemmed from drives denied their natural release.

The unconscious and free association

If the laws of energy conservation applied to the mind then new ideas and feeling had to come from somewhere. Freud observed the power of unblocking 'unconscious' forces after visiting the French neurologist Charcot, who used hypnosis to cure hysterical disorders such as fits or mutism. Freud initially found hypnosis and suggestion successful with many of his patients but the results were often only temporary. He began to encourage them, under hypnosis, to recall the events leading up to their illness and concluded that traumatic memories were often the cause.

More importantly he concluded that his patients were unaware of much of their 'thinking'—that some mental processes were *unconscious*. The harder one tried to become aware of them, the harder it got. Freud found a way round this by developing his technique of 'free association'. He encouraged his patient to stop *trying* to remember and instead say whatever came into their mind. From these 'random' remarks, supplemented by recounting dreams, repressed thoughts 'leaked out' in obscure ways. You can almost see him imagining steam driving pistons! The analyst used his own unconscious to 'listen' to these remarks, detecting patterns and thereby directing the patient towards the source of their troubles. Hence a 'Freudian slip' is when someone's true thoughts slip out by mistake. Freud became obsessed with the need not to interfere with this free association. The 'blank screen' therapist should reveal nothing about themselves, often sitting behind the patient and never directly answering questions or giving reassurance. It is hard to imagine, looking at the picture of Freud's consulting room (Figure 5), and knowing about the controversies that surrounded him throughout his life, how he could ever believe he was a blank screen.

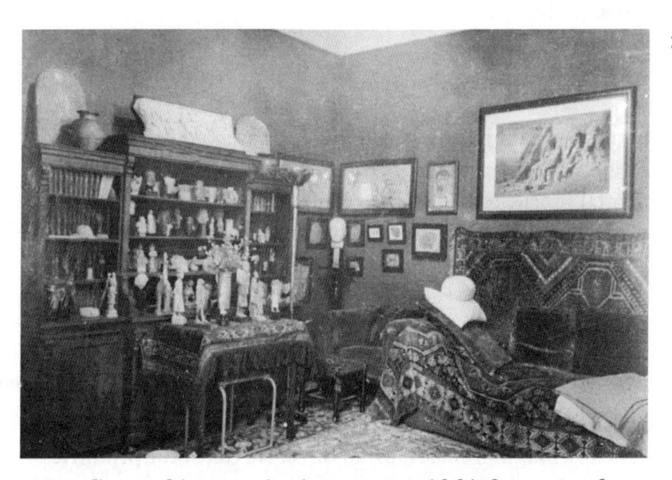

5. Freud's consulting room in Vienna *c.*1910 with his famous couch.

Nineteenth-century bourgeois Vienna was a very inhibited society, particularly for upper-class women. Not surprisingly many of the unconscious conflicts that Freud uncovered were sexual. Initially he believed that his patients had been sexually abused, but in a dramatic reversal he came to believe that these reports were more often fantasies and wish-fulfilments. He proposed his theory of infantile sexuality—that even very small children have strong 'sexual' feelings about their parents. This, of course, caused uproar, and in many circles still does. The language is over-blown, but the ideas do help make some sense of the intense and powerful dynamics in families. The Oedipus Complex is probably its most famous consequence. Freud proposed that at about 3 years old the young boy desires his mother intensely and views his father as a frightening rival for her affections (based on the Greek myth of Oedipus who killed his father and married his mother). Put so, it seems pretty unhelpful, but it is an insightful way to understand how some people never learn to share important relationships. In the process of striving for exclusive intimacy, they destroy what they most want. It made sense of many of the patients Freud saw, as it does today.

Ego, id, and superego

Freud originally believed that the conscious mind was entirely rational in contrast to more primitive, less logical, unconscious mental processes. This may explain some of his exaggerated terminology. However, he was struck by the savage, punitive consciences of some of his patients. How could something as noble as conscience (Freud was a strictly moral individual himself) drive a patient to suicide through guilt? His solution was to describe the conscience as derived from both conscious thoughts and also powerful unconscious remnants of parental and social demands. His map of the mind expanded from two areas (unconscious and conscious) to three. He called the primitive unconscious the id (the 'it'), the conscious mind the ego (the 'I'), and the conscience the superego (literally the 'over I'). All are now part of everyday speech.

Defence mechanisms

Early psychoanalysis was about enabling the patient to discover repressed conflicts. Initially, Freud thought this was sufficient. However, as analyses became longer and more complex, analysts encountered 'resistance' where patients appeared to block change using various psychological defence mechanisms. For Freud the most troublesome resistance was when patients kept falling in love with him (or at the very least seeing him as a father figure). At one level this helped—patients who like you will work hard and do what you ask. He called these feelings 'transference', because he thought they were *transferred* from important figures in the patient's past life and he found they made exploring free associations difficult. However, from initially thinking of transference as a problem, Freud started to exploit it in analysis. This 'analysis of defence mechanisms' became an essential part of treatment.

There were many blind alleys in Freud's work, which is no surprise in someone who wrote so much. He made us aware of the power of unacknowledged thoughts and how the past can continue to haunt lives. Even more important, he showed that a brave attempt to confront and understand the origins of problems (not simply to offer support and comfort) although initially quite painful and demanding can lead to liberation and relief. He also (against his own wishes, no doubt) showed how an honestly entered and reflective human relationship can itself serve as a tool for recovery in mental illness.

Freud was a pessimist (writing after the carnage of the First World War) and never promised happiness. Psychoanalysis, he wrote, would 'convert your hysterical misery into normal human unhappiness', and his highest ambition was for a patient to be able 'to work and to love'. No more, no less. The rigidity and grandiosity of many of his successors has tarnished his reputation. His claims to have been a scientist are questionable and his treatment, psychoanalysis, is under siege for its failure to provide adequate evidence of its effectiveness. However, he has probably contributed as much to understanding and tolerance in the care of the mentally ill as any other individual. His insistence on taking the patient's past seriously and his vivid metaphors for mental processes are readily grasped by therapists and patients alike. They have formed the basis for a humane working relationship for which he deserves more credit than is currently his lot.

Jung

Freud collected about him a glittering band of followers—all men and all Jewish. As often with such creative groups there were conflicts, and splits. Several took the approach in differing directions and their influences have waxed and waned. Carl-Gustav Jung (1875–1961), the first non-Jewish member of the circle, had the most lasting impact. While Freud called himself a 'Godless Jew' with little sense of the spiritual or transcendent, Jung's theories were more mystical. They included a racial unconscious with 'archetypes' (symbolic figures which we all share) and an emphasis on the importance of opposites in our personalities, especially how a 'shadow self' develops from those aspects we refuse to acknowledge. Many believe Jung suffered a brief psychotic breakdown himself and drew on some of these deeply irrational experiences. Unlike Freud, he believed that therapy could aim beyond symptom resolution to promote deep personal fulfilment, and his approach is popular with those who work with very ill patients and in creative circles. Jung originated the idea of *introvert* and *extrovert* personality types which are now in daily usage by millions who have probably never heard of him.

Psychodynamic psychotherapy

Psychoanalysis was closely associated with Jewish practitioners in its infancy and became a target for Nazi persecution in the 1930s.

Analysts had to leave and most moved to the USA, England, and South America where they came to have an enormous influence on psychiatry—much more than in their native German-speaking countries.

The Second World War put extra demands on psychoanalysts who then turned their attention to traumatized soldiers and, more surprisingly, army management. Out of this arose group analysis and group therapies where patients were treated in small groups of 5–8, thereby benefiting from solidarity and support as well as insight. Group work generated the therapeutic community (see Chapter 3), where analytical and psychological insights are applied to running a ward (rather than just individual treatments). This informal, communal approach (with staff and patients sharing daily tasks) was called 'sociotherapy' and has become a standard feature of modern psychiatric practice, drug rehabilitation units, and some prisons.

The seeming endlessness of classic psychoanalysis (three to five sessions a week for several years) has been strongly criticized. It is prohibitively expensive (and therefore exclusive), and many believed that shorter therapies would focus the mind better and improve outcomes. Short-term therapies are now more the norm, with weekly sessions of an hour over three to six months. Interpersonal Therapy (IPT) focuses on relationships and Cognitive Analytical Therapy (CAT) uses specific exercises like letter writing and prescription of homework as part of the treatment. While still maintaining strict professional boundaries, therapists are increasingly more active.

These are usually called 'psychodynamic' psychotherapies because they attribute importance to dynamic interactions between the past and the present and between conscious and unconscious processes. The individual's life story, 'their narrative', is central to understanding and resolving problems. All require the therapist to hold back from giving too much direct advice so that the patient can, with guidance, find their own solutions. These therapies can be used in parallel with other psychiatric treatments (antidepressants, hospital care, etc.). There is no strict ideological opposition.

Non-specific factors in psychotherapy

Most psychodynamic psychotherapists are intensely loyal to their specific model. Unfortunately, the evidence is against them. There is depressingly little research into psychodynamic psychotherapies (unlike Cognitive Behavioural Therapy (CBT)), but what there is makes interesting reading. Experienced therapists who follow their training closely are effective and they do much better than novices, or those who apply their model loosely. However, *which* model doesn't seem to matter so much—they are all about equally effective. Most of this research confirms the crucial importance of establishing a good therapeutic relationship.

In short, the qualities of a good therapist transcend the different psychotherapy types and the essential ingredients have been identified. They are *accurate empathy* (the therapist must really understand what the patient is going through, it is not enough just to feel sorry for them), *unconditional regard* (the therapist has to like and respect the patient, you cannot do therapy with someone you really dislike), and *non-possessive warmth* (the therapist must be able to show warmth and support without making the patient feel beholden to them). These insights are particularly useful in psychiatric practice. Matching patients and therapists really does matter—none of us can get on with absolutely everyone. Work with violent or sexual offenders, for instance, requires particularly tolerant and forgiving therapists.

Existential and experimental psychotherapies

Several schools of psychotherapy utilize psychodynamic psychotherapy techniques without accepting the theory. Existential psychotherapy, as its name suggests, makes no assumptions about what people 'should be like' but focuses on helping the patient express their own identity. Existential psychotherapies have become more popular as society becomes less rigid and conformist.

Freud's patients usually shared their family's and society's expectations and became distressed when they could not meet them. In the early 21st century we are more likely to experience aimlessness and emptiness rather than guilt at not living up to expectations. As alienation and confusion have become more frequent complaints, psychotherapies have become more structured, providing boundaries and containment.

These more here-and-now therapies blend imperceptibly into the personal growth movement. It can be difficult sometimes to decide whether a personal growth group or an encounter group are *treatments* to reduce suffering or *exercises* to increase personal happiness and fulfilment. Perhaps it doesn't matter what the purpose is so much as who gets it. There can be little doubt that depressed and demoralized psychiatric patients benefit greatly from such activities, which lift morale and self-esteem. In treating self-harming young women, addressing self-esteem directly is often the most effective intervention.

Psychodynamic psychotherapies are currently under attack in psychiatry for inadequate research to show that they work. Also, the requirement of a personal training therapy and persisting supervision can compromise objectivity and smacks of a 'cult' rather than a profession. There is some research into short-term dynamic therapies and the results are generally good. However, more detailed studies to identify which bits are effective, and which redundant, are needed. The opportunity for such research may even have passed. Many of the core features of psychodynamic psychotherapy are now so routine (as in the Type A and B treatments) that their specific contributions may be difficult to isolate and evaluate.

The strength of criticism is not surprising as psychoanalysis really did oversell itself shamelessly in America (North and South). Between 1940 and 1970 it virtually drove all other thinking out of mental health care—most people thought that a psychiatrist *was* a psychoanalyst. Psychotic patients, for whom analysis had little to offer, were neglected, as were the basic skills of diagnosis and treatment. Critics accused American psychiatry in this period, with its high status and expanding workforce, of simply turning its back on the severely mentally ill and on science. President Kennedy tried to refocus the profession in the early 1960s but without success, and it required the pharmacological revolution in the succeeding decade to achieve it. A more scientific and self-critical psychiatry, obliged to establish itself with hard won research data, has taken its revenge on psychoanalysis (and some would say is now beginning to exhibit the same hubris—Chapter 6).

The newer psychotherapies and counselling

The last forty years have seen the development of a whole series of new psychotherapies that are radically different. They pay far less attention to understanding the past. The therapists are usually more directive—they give instructions and opinions, not just further encouragement to the patient to continue reflecting. Many involve specific exercises and 'homework' that is reviewed in sessions. They last months not years and reject the mystique common to psychodynamic therapists.

Person-centred (often called Rogerian) counselling is one such approach. The distinction between counselling and psychotherapy is variable and unclear. Counselling is often offered at times of personal crisis to people we would not usually consider as 'ill', hence the use of 'client' rather than 'patient'. Its aims are more modest than formal therapy. It emphasizes the characteristics of a good therapist to provide a 'safe space' for the client to explore their distress. Here the therapist really is non-directive.

They rarely give opinions or advise the patient but often simply repeat back the client's last phrase as encouragement to continue reflecting. Counselling is a skill highly prized by many mental health professionals and clearly valued by patients.

Family and systems therapies and crisis intervention

Family therapies are particularly important in the treatment of psychiatrically ill children. Family therapists do not consider the family to blame for the illness (see Chapter 5), but it may be impossible for a patient to get better unless the whole family changes its way of responding. In anorexia nervosa, for instance, a family may have become so anxious about their daughter's condition that they cannot allow her the freedom to take necessary personal risks and so to grow and mature. They may need help to back off and contain their anxiety. Sometimes the same can occur with adult patients where family therapy often helps couples address a destructive pattern in their relationship. Family therapy usually relies on a 'systems' approach where the whole family is the focus, not the individual members.

'Behavioural family management' is used to help families of schizophrenia patients. Breakdowns are more frequent if patients live in highly emotional families—especially where marked by tension or criticism. It may be very difficult for the family to avoid this, so the treatment identifies flash-points in the relationships and helps find alternative solutions (e.g. going into another room rather than arguing back). Relapse rates are substantially reduced, but the treatment is protracted and it is difficult.

Crisis therapy is in here with systems therapies because it deals with immediate problems. You don't have to dig around in crisis or family therapy to unearth issues. They're all there right in front of you. Crisis therapy is dramatic, ultra short-term, and handles strong emotions, usually with only limited attention to their origins. While the family therapies are generally well established, there remain doubts about crisis therapy. Indeed, research shows that routine crisis debriefing after trauma can even make things worse, and it is now actively discouraged in UK psychiatry. Presumably it interferes with the healthy processes of forgetting and moving on.

Behaviour therapy

Behaviour therapy principles are about as different from psychodynamic psychotherapy as it is possible to be. They are based on learning theory and make a virtue of removing 'consciousness' from the equation—change is explained by reflex learning. The psychologist B. F. Skinner developed Pavlov's observation of conditioned reflexes in his dogs to train rats in complex behaviours. He did this simply by rewarding the behaviour he wanted or 'punishing' the behaviour he wanted to stop. Behaviour is 'shaped' in small steps, one at a time ('operant conditioning'). Behaviour therapy is unique in that the subject neither needs to agree to, or even know, what is going on—the learning is entirely unconscious.

Behaviour therapy can be staggeringly effective—think how easy it is to ride a bike and yet you probably have never 'consciously' learnt. You just tried it and each time it started to go wrong your body compensated, and now you are supremely skilled. Behaviour therapy works like that. It has proved particularly effective in treatments for individuals with learning disabilities and with children. A simple example of operant conditioning is the bell-and-pad system for nocturnal enuresis (bed wetting). A bell rings as soon as the pad gets wet, waking the patient. Over time he starts to wake up when his (it is usually his) bladder is full, as that sensation becomes associated with the bell and being woken. This successful treatment is widely and successfully used despite evidence that the condition may be predominantly genetic.

Behaviour therapy is extensively used for phobias and for obsessive compulsive disorders. The patient is gradually exposed to the feared stimulus (e.g. dirt rubbed onto the hand for someone with obsessions about germs) while restricting immediate avoidance (not allowing them to wash it off) while monitoring anxiety to ensure it remains tolerable. In practice behaviour therapists still take detailed histories because, without a good therapeutic relationship, patients drop out of treatment.

Cognitive behavioural therapy

Cognitive behavioural therapy could equally be considered a sophisticated extension of behaviour therapy, or an adaptation of psychodynamic psychotherapy. It lies somewhere between the two. It was developed by the psychoanalytically trained American psychiatrist Aaron Beck who noticed that some of his patients did not improve. These were generally people who prized mastery of their symptoms rather than understanding them. His investigations convinced him that it was unconscious and pathological *thoughts* more than feelings that were trapping his patients. He developed a therapy to enable patients to identify 'automatic negative thoughts' (self-critical, self-defeating beliefs and conclusions) and to train them in how to directly challenge and contradict them.

His method emphasized 'Socratic Dialogue'. The Greek philosopher Socrates believed that all you needed to learn the truth was to keep asking the right questions and the answers eventually arose from within. So when the patient expresses a pathological doubt—e.g. 'I got it wrong at work today. There's no future for me'—the therapist asks them to explain it: 'OK, you got it wrong but explain to me why there is no hope.' He contrasts the thoughts with the reality of the situation—'Explain how it is that you're still being promoted at work then, despite these mistakes?' CBT is now an essential part of psychiatric practice and training and is standard in the treatments of depression and anxiety. It is increasingly used in a whole range of disorders including schizophrenia with intractable hallucinations or delusions and in physical disorders with a significant psychological component.

Self-help

It may not be psychiatry, but the self-help movement (Alcoholics Anonymous, Weight Watchers, The Depression Alliance) all use what they have learnt from psychotherapy, and more. For accurate empathy and unconditional regard—who better than someone who has been through it? Who less likely to condemn? Non-possessive warmth—what better source than shared suffering and real fellow-feeling? Self-help groups constitute a folk movement of our times; they relieve distress and isolation and reduce stigma. Self-help books, apps, and web-based learning are increasingly available for common disorders such as anxiety and depression. It is too early to judge their lasting impact, but they certainly get the popular vote.

After 200 years of psychiatry, it seems strange for psychotherapy to be restricted to its own short chapter. Can it really be considered separate from psychiatry or psychiatry separate from it? Psychotherapy has been a defining characteristic of the psychiatric craft: as central to psychiatry as operating is to a surgeon or delivering babies to an obstetrician. Asylum doctors of 150 years ago spent time talking with distressed patients to bring understanding, comfort, and relief. In the second half of the 20th century this personal relationship was why most staff came into the profession. Yet into the 21st century they are increasingly considered as parallel activities. Is psychiatry changing fundamentally? Will they come together again or pursue increasingly independent paths? Some of the forces driving these changes will occupy us in Chapter 7.

Chapter 5
Psychiatry under attack—inside and out

Psychiatry has always been controversial—there never was a 'Golden Age' of peace and tranquillity when everybody admired it. You possibly bought this book following some discussion about its rights and wrongs. Because it deals with the mind, and because psychiatrists can override our wishes, it invariably evokes some suspicion and fear. Nor is this simply down to ignorance, that if people knew more they wouldn't worry. There are very real questions to be asked about psychiatry—both about its legitimacy as a medical speciality, and about how it is practised. All modern medicine generates ethical challenges and controversies and psychiatry has had more than its fair share (Chapter 6). This chapter will focus on the contradictions *inherent* in psychiatry, those that stem from its very nature, rather than its implementation.

Mind–body dualism

The French philosopher René Descartes (1596–1650) is often blamed for how we separate the mind from the body in Western thought, often referred to as 'Cartesian dualism'. His 'cogito ergo sum' ('I think therefore I am') is snappy and memorable; it expresses his scepticism that we could know about the material world with any certainty. Why has he been singled out when this question has exercised most philosophers? He didn't *invent* the problem of the mind; he simply put it more memorably and it remains essentially unresolved 350 years later. What the mind is, and how it interacts with the material world, are still mysteries. Most of us *do* think there is a difference, and most of us accept that there *is* an interaction. We have to believe we can directly influence the material world (e.g. I can trust that I really can move my hand forward and type in my computer). We also need to believe that we can know the minds of others (e.g. I'm sure that you will go to the library or hand in your essay). Without these beliefs we would effectively be paralysed.

The mind–body question is unavoidable in psychiatry. The relationship between the mind and the brain is *the* issue. It would be simple if psychiatry were just about 'brain diseases' in the way that nephrology is about kidney diseases or cardiology is about heart diseases, but it is not. Psychiatry concerns 'mental' illnesses. While many mental illnesses clearly involve disorders of the brain (e.g. disturbances in transmitter chemicals between cells in depression and schizophrenia) others do not. In addition not all brain diseases are mental illnesses. Multiple sclerosis and Parkinson's disease are brain diseases, but neurologists, not psychiatrists, treat them and we call them neurological illnesses, not mental illnesses. Such neurological disorders, like many other physical illnesses, often *cause* psychiatric problems. Many psychiatric disorders include physical symptoms (e.g. tiredness and pain), just as physical disorders include psychiatric symptoms (e.g. depression, anxiety, and even hallucinations).

In short, mental illnesses have their *main* disturbances in thoughts, feelings, and behaviour (Chapter 1). A common misconception is that physical diseases have physical causes and cures while mental diseases have mental causes and cures. Illnesses can have physical causes and even physical cures (e.g. a depression caused by Parkinson's disease and treated by antidepressants) and still be 'mental illnesses'. The division is pragmatic and philosophically unsatisfying. It is based on the *main* disturbances and on the *skills* needed to help. 'Mental disorders are brain disorders' was a popular slogan with some psychiatrists and patient groups in the 1990s. Its purpose was to emphasize the similarity between mental and physical illnesses, thereby hopefully reducing stigma and blame. Despite admirable goals, it is an over-simplification and failed to fully convince. Psychiatry has struggled with this ambiguity in two main battlegrounds.

Nature versus nurture: do families cause mental illness?

Whether we're tall or short, good at sport or hopeless at it, most of us believe depends on a mixture of our genes (the biological potential we are born with) and our upbringing (our diet, exercise regime, even the sort of school we went to). Nothing controversial there. But the moment we touch on psychology or behaviour disputes arise. Is IQ inherited or could everyone do just as well with the same opportunities? Is personality or criminality something we're born with or can we change it? Can we avoid depression by healthy living? Few issues polarize us as much as how malleable we believe human nature is. These disagreements are not just dry, academic discussions but fuel (and are fuelled by) political and social beliefs reflecting fundamentally different worldviews.

Psychiatry was originally very much at home in the 'nature' camp—mental illnesses ran in families and so were inherited weaknesses. Our role was to ameliorate them, making life bearable while hoping for a speedy recovery. Freud and his followers changed all that, shifting the balance to 'nurture'. Psychoanalysis is firmly based on the belief that what happens to us in early life, and the memories of those experiences, are the *cause* of many illnesses. Even more convincing, Freud showed that addressing those memories could *cure* some mental illnesses. So an individual's personal history wasn't just the context for understanding their illness but possibly its origin.

Psychoanalysis dominated psychiatric thinking and training from the 1940s to the 1970s. Its attraction to the Americas should come as no surprise. These are societies established by those fleeing the Europe of fixed social orders and aristocracies. Those moving west rejected this resignation, seeking the opportunity to shape their own futures. Hence the attraction of a psychology that enshrined this capacity for growth, where the individual could overcome personal adversity to forge their own destiny. The importance of nurture and personal experience was strengthened by the experiences with battle trauma in both world wars (Chapter 3). The revelation of the eugenic and racist policies of Nazi Germany (including the liquidation of 'genetically inferior' psychiatric patients) finally guaranteed nurture's moral superiority.

An attraction of nurture is that it promises a greater likelihood of cure. If mental illnesses are essentially *caused* by relationships, then they should be curable by relationships (i.e. psychotherapy). A risk with this view is its potential for blame—in particular blaming parents. Freud himself quickly realized this when he began to suspect that the reported sexual abuse by parents was not the trauma underlying neurosis but a projected fantasy. The German psychopathologist Jaspers pointed out that, while understanding the personal relevance of symptoms was essential, it did not explain what *caused* the illness. Such fine distinctions have not, however, generally characterized this debate.

The origins of schizophrenia

This controversy has raged most fiercely over the origins of schizophrenia. Schizophrenia had always been observed to run in families and sometimes those families could seem 'odd' (often eccentric or withdrawn). They also often exhibited strained or intensely over-involved relationships. As schizophrenia is expressed in thinking and relating, a causal link with early upbringing was obviously plausible. Family life is, after all, conducted through thinking, feeling, and relating as it equips the growing child with skills in these areas. Applying psychoanalytical practice to schizophrenia (which Freud actively opposed) generated speculative theories, some of which remain influential.

The 'schizophrenogenic mother'

The most notorious (and probably most damaging) theory was of the cold, hostile, and yet controlling parent—the 'schizophrenogenic mother'. This was proposed by an analyst, Frieda Fromm-Reichmann, who worked in long-term intensive psychoanalysis with hospitalized schizophrenia patients in the USA. Joanna Greenberg described her treatment in a best-selling autobiographical novel *I Never Promised You a Rose-Garden.*

The schizophrenogenic mother was a powerful, but cold and rejecting, figure who bound the patient close to her, preventing the growth of healthy independence and sense of self. Schizophrenia was consequently understood as a disorder of 'ego-development' with weak personal boundaries (hence the confusion of internal and external experiences in hallucinations). Fromm-Reichmann's conclusions are preposterous by current standards. She based them solely on patients' reports, rarely meeting or interviewing the mothers. Despite its early rejection within the profession, the conviction lives on that faulty parenting can 'cause' schizophrenia. This has led to endless self-blame by parents and, in some circumstances, rejection and exclusion by mental health professionals.

The 'double-bind'

The 'double-bind' is one of the most enduring of these theories. An anthropologist, Gregory Bateson, proposed that it was persistent, logically faulty, and contradictory communication with a child that prevented it forming a proper sense of itself and its relationships to the external world. Bateson's idea arose from the mathematical law that a number designating a series of numbers could not itself be a member of that series—it was of a 'logically different order'. He argued that similar, logically different, levels existed in communication. When we send messages to each other one part of the message (often in an obscure, non-verbal manner) indicated how the main message should be interpreted. He called these 'meta-communications' (i.e. communications about communication). Typically meta-communications were emotional and non-verbal and became strongly held family assumptions (e.g. 'mother can only love her children and always feel positive about them').

Bateson called it a double-bind when the non-verbal message and verbal message contradicted each other (e.g. an obviously angry mother saying she didn't mind at all that the child had broken a glass and holding her arms out for an embrace). A double-bind required three components: a clear simple message, a contradictory meta-communication, and a family prohibition on the contradiction being acknowledged. It is this family culture of denying the contradiction that is most pathological. After all, all families give contradictory and confusing messages. 'Double-bind' is used loosely for any contradictory communication, but Bateson's construction was much more specific.

These theories are now conclusively discredited. Independent researchers listened to tapes of families with and without schizophrenia and rated the occurrence of double-binds, and interviewed families and rated them for coldness, hostility, over-involvement, etc. Differences were simply not found. Adoption studies, however, delivered the *coup de grâce* to these ideas. Children of schizophrenic mothers adopted away at birth to healthy families developed schizophrenia when they grew up just as frequently as if they had been brought up with their biological mother. Similarly, twins adopted away at birth to different families demonstrated the same established rates for both becoming ill in identical as non-identical twins. Of course none of these risks are absolute and upbringing and environment do have significant effects.

While family influence as the sole *cause* of schizophrenia has been conclusively dismissed, it remains relevant for the *course* of the illness. Patients in highly emotional families break down more often. It could, of course, be because families with more severely ill members become more stressed and stressful (see Chapter 4). However, training families to respond less emotionally does reduce the rate of breakdown, so such 'high expressed emotion' probably does have a direct effect.

Social and peer-group pressure

While the idea of families as the cause of mental illness has been displaced, wider social influences have received increasing recognition. For example, the rise in eating disorders (anorexia nervosa and bulimia) has spread from the West, closely tracking the cultural ideal of thinness in women. The epidemic of self-harm (particularly overdosing and cutting in younger women) is clearly affected by group norms and expectations. Local outbreaks can often be linked to specific events such as suicide attempts in TV soap operas. Alcohol and drug use are highly variable both between and within countries and the influence of group expectations is striking.

Evolutionary psychology

The nature–nurture argument has recently been revived by the rise of evolutionary psychology. A more sophisticated understanding of Darwinian evolution (survival of the fittest) has led to theories about the possible evolutionary value of some of the traits underlying psychiatric disorders. A simplistic Darwinian understanding would predict that mental illnesses should lower survival and ought to die out. 'Inclusive fitness' stresses that evolutionary value depends on whether their *offspring* are more likely to survive, rather than the *individual* itself.

Some evolutionary advantages for mental illnesses have been hypothesized from ethological games-theory. This understands the benefits or drawbacks of any behaviour as depending on the behaviour of other group members. So depression might be seen as a safe response to 'defeat' in a hierarchical group because it withdraws the individual, thus protecting them from conflict while they recover. Conversely, mania, with its expansiveness and increased sexual activity, is proposed as a response to success in a hierarchical tussle, which promotes the propagation of that individual's genes. Behaviours resembling depression and hypomania are clearly evident in primates as they move up and down the pecking order that dominates their lives.

Schizophrenia, with its social isolation and withdrawal, has been speculatively proposed to protect from infectious diseases and epidemics, or even as adaptive to remote habitats with limited food resources and sparse populations. Evolutionary psychology is still highly controversial as some gender specific theories appear to excuse a male-orientated, exploitative worldview.

Why do families blame themselves?

If family theories have been so roundly discredited why devote so much space to them here? It is because they continue to exercise a remarkably powerful hold over us despite the evidence against them. Parents seem to have an endless capacity to blame themselves for what happens to their children (and perhaps children to blame their parents). It appears that we perhaps *need* to believe it. Evolutionary psychologists say that parents need to have an exaggerated view of their importance in order to invest the years and years it takes to bring up children. We have evolved belief systems to explain to ourselves our biologically programmed behaviour. The belief is a mechanism for sustaining our attention to our biological task. It is a product of our behaviour, rather than a cause of it.

The downside of this is guilt and blame. We believe we have failed if things go badly. Even when therapists insist emphatically that no one is to blame, families still feel blamed. 'If only we weren't so over-involved he would have stayed well.' 'Other families manage better otherwise how would you know what to advise?' For some families feeling responsible, despite the guilt, is preferable as it carries the promise that there may be *something* they can do to make it better. More fatalistic cultures seem less prone to such blame; high expressed emotion has been shown to be less common in India than in Europe.

The anti-psychiatry movement

These arguments over mind and brain and nature and nurture erupted into the most sustained and celebrated 'external' onslaught on psychiatry in the 1960s and 1970s. The mental hospital scandals of the early 1960s and publication of Erving Goffman's *Asylums* had prepared the ground for a devastating attack by a group dubbed 'the anti-psychiatrists'. They went beyond criticisms of psychiatry's practices and failures to an assault on its very legitimacy.

The anti-psychiatry message was that psychiatry did not need improving, it needed scrapping. At its best psychiatry was confused and confusing, and at its worst an instrument of social oppression masquerading as a benign medical practice. Three charismatic authors came to personify the movement. Two were practising psychiatrists. Their books became campus bibles in the widespread student unrest of the late 1960s and early 1970s.

Thomas Szasz, a Hungarian immigrant to the USA, argued in his 1961 book *The Myth of Mental Illness* that 'mental illnesses' were simply fabrications to deny socially deviant individuals their legal rights. He believed that the absence of a measurable physical marker (such as blood sugar levels in diabetes) meant that mental illnesses were not true illnesses but merely social constructs. He argued vigorously against involuntary treatment, for the complete separation of psychiatry from the state, and the abolition of the insanity defence. Those judged mentally ill should be treated equally and held accountable for their actions, psychotic individuals could refuse treatment and go to prison if they break the law. His extreme libertarian standpoint and opposition to compulsion may reflect his childhood under Soviet occupation.

Michel Foucault was a French philosopher who believed that the concept of mental illness was an aberration of the post-Enlightenment age. He objected to the classification of identities, arguing that the existence of *madness* did not entail the identity of *madman*. His book *Madness and Civilisation* conceived of psychiatric practice as repressive and controlling, rather than curing and liberating. His work had enormous influence in continental Europe (most evident in Basaglia's reforms in Italy). His writing is dense and difficult to absorb, and he is more often quoted than read.

The most accessible and influential of the anti-psychiatrists was R. D. Laing. A Glaswegian psychoanalyst with a brilliant mind and lucid prose style, he turned the psychiatric world upside down with a series of best-selling books. An original and impulsive man, his views changed throughout his career, and like Freud he didn't stop to explain his changes. His first, and most influential, book was *The Divided Self: An Existential Study in Sanity and Madness* (1960). He called his position 'existential phenomenology', proposing that the delusional thinking of the schizophrenia patient was simply a different take on the world. This thinking could be challenging, but it was essentially creative and, with enough imagination and moral courage, could be understood. However, these different worldviews threaten our security so we seek to deny them by imposing a diagnosis and 'pathologizing' them.

The book is filled with vivid descriptions of patients Laing had treated, accompanied with the most moving and imaginative interpretations of their dilemma. The impression given of psychosis by *The Divided Self* was of a tormented but heroic individual who communicated vivid, authentic experiences, only to be met by a fearful and mean-spirited rejection. Although he did not deny patients' suffering, his was essentially a romantic view of madness which, ironically, increased recruitment into psychiatry while attacking it. Like Szasz, Laing never called himself an anti-psychiatrist and continued to treat patients, albeit in unorthodox ways.

Laing's second 'phase' was his belief that families contributed to schizophrenia by denying the emerging identity of their child. *Sanity, Madness and the Family: Families of Schizophrenics*, with Aaron Esterson, cast schizophrenia as a response to repressive and rejecting parenting. This includes echoes of the double-bind and schizophrenogenic mother, and a film inspired by it (*Family Life*, 1971) struck an international chord. Laing's third phase was inspired by his extensive experimentation with LSD. *The Politics of Experience and the Bird of Paradise* was published in 1967. In this he considered psychosis as a psychedelic voyage of discovery in which the boundaries of perception were widened, and consciousness expanded ('a break through rather than a breakdown').

Laing was an improbable candidate for such an influential role. Starting as an army psychiatrist, he became a celebrity psychoanalyst. His personal life was turbulent, with several marriages and many children, experimenting with Eastern mysticism, and drinking to excess. As a lecturer he ranged from the inspirational to the frankly intoxicated and unintelligible. He had enormous ability to galvanize anti-establishment feeling—after a lecture to students in Tokyo in 1969 they went off and set fire to the university administration building! (Figure 6.) He remained a radical until his death, aged 62, surprising all who knew him by

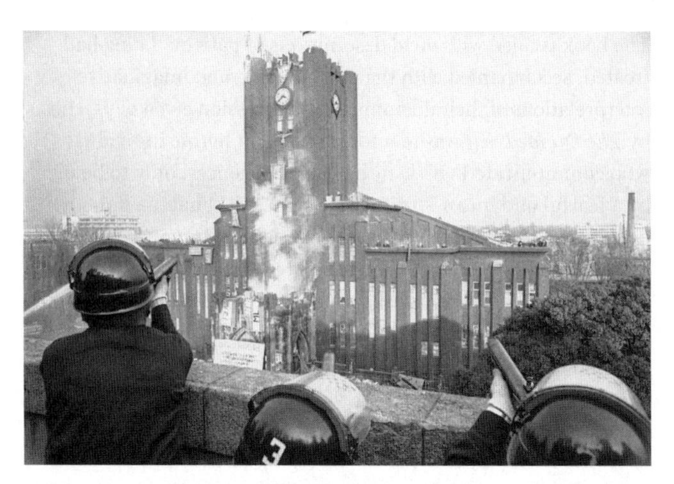

6. The remains of the psychiatry department in Tokyo after students burnt it down following R. D. Laing's lecture in 1969.

collapsing in the outrageously bourgeois activity of playing tennis on the French Riviera.

Radical and Post Psychiatry

The contradictions inherent in psychiatry which generated the anti-psychiatry movement in the 1960s and 1970s have not gone away. Mind and brain, freedom and coercion, the right to be different (perhaps even the *duty* to be different), nature and nurture remain issues for us still. Many ex-patient groups are militantly anti-psychiatric, calling themselves 'survivors' rather than patients, clients, or service users. In Germany and Holland the state contributes to hostels and crash pads for individuals who have 'escaped' routine mental health services. The most high-profile anti-psychiatry group is probably the Church of Scientology. While much of their focus is on controversial treatments such as brain surgery and ECT (Chapter 6), they are roundly critical of the whole endeavour.

Overall, however, there is now much less concerted opposition to psychiatry as a discipline. This may, in part, be due to a somewhat exaggerated faith in the rapid expansion of 'biological' explanations and an optimism that genetic and genomic advances will soon render the whole issue historic. Radical psychiatry does, however, persist in groups of professionals agitating for a more human, less technical approach and a reining in of over-prescribing. The term 'Post Psychiatrists' refers to a view that the benefits of scientism, and in particular bio-medicine, have been exaggerated and a more equal personalized approach with less focus on certainty and diagnosis is urgently needed. However, while there is less conceptual opposition to psychiatry, there is no shortage of disquiet about various aspects of its practice. We turn to these in Chapter 6.

Chapter 6
Open to abuse

Controversies in psychiatric practice

The very nature of psychiatric practice lays it open to potential misuse and abuse. It involves a highly unequal power relationship with dependent and vulnerable patients whose complaints can so easily be dismissed as 'part of the illness'. Add to this the subjective nature of a diagnostic process which relies on an assessment of motives and mental state with no concrete indicators of the disease. Our history doesn't inspire that much confidence either. There have been shameful episodes of political abuse, some hare-brained theories, and treatments that appear now both dangerous and barbaric. The very visibility of modern-day psychiatry (out from behind the institutions' walls), plus a well-informed public and a greater willingness to admit if things go wrong, are probably our most reliable safeguards against abuses. Psychiatry has also now, thankfully, fully engaged with evidence-based medicine—facts and figures take precedence over theories and opinion. So while we focus in this chapter on what it can get wrong, let's not forget that it more often gets it right and that progress has been enormous.

In the public imagination psychiatry's threat lies in its immense power. The evil psychiatrist is portrayed in films manipulating the minds of his hapless victim for his own ends, taking pleasure in subjugating the distressed and suggestible. The terrifying Dr Hannibal Lecter in *Silence of the Lambs* uses his immense skill to read his victims' minds to trap and exploit them. In other films psychiatrists develop megalomaniacal delusions of using their power to rule the world.

There have undoubtedly been cases where psychiatrists, convinced of their own infallibility, have wreaked havoc. Experiments with altering gender identity to confirm that it was socially determined was one extreme example. The craze to remove sources of infection in teeth and bowels that were deemed the cause of mental illness, and the wholesale use of lobotomy in the 1940s and early 1950s, were others. However most of psychiatry's excesses have stemmed from the very opposite, from psychiatrists' turning to well-intentioned but ever more desperate interventions from their frustration over not being able to help very distressed patients.

This relationship is changing. Professions are no longer so powerful and unaccountable. Deference and respect for authority have reduced everywhere. Risks now may come less from professional isolation and arrogance than from excessive social compliance. Monitoring psychiatrists may be only half of the job—we need to keep a wary eye on the multinational drug companies, governments, and pressure groups who can manipulate psychiatry.

Old sins

Like all of medicine, psychiatry's history includes what would now appear dangerous and even barbaric treatments. Before leaping to judgement, we should imagine how life was then, when early and sudden death was a constant threat and excruciating pain had to be endured sometimes indefinitely. There were few certainties and even fewer effective treatments. What doctors were willing to do two centuries ago, and what patients were prepared to endure, have to be judged against quite different standards. Folk treatments of the mad were also far from innocuous, despite our tendency to romanticize pre-industrial societies. Disabled individuals may have been accepted and occasionally revered, but the disturbed were more frequently excluded (which often meant death) or mistreated.

Early psychiatrists used the routine, often painful, medical treatments of their time including bleeding, purging, and cupping (attaching hot cups to the back to 'draw out' toxins, curiously fashionable again in health clubs). The early asylums moved away from these, emphasizing moral treatments (Chapter 2), although various desperate measures were tried to calm agitated patients. These included cold baths (still used well into the 20th century) and various devices which simply exhausted the patient, such as the notorious 'whirling chair' (Figure 7). However, the major sins of the asylum era were those of neglect—restraint rather than attention, undignified and humiliating conditions rather than active abuse (Figure 8).

Long-term fluctuating illnesses with no effective treatments are particularly prone to accumulate far-fetched theories and interventions. This is a mixture of desperation and pure chance. A spontaneous recovery coinciding with some random treatment can establish its reputation. There was a vogue for removing otherwise healthy organs in the mentally ill (though not only in the mentally ill) in the late 19th century because they were thought to be the sites of 'sepsis' (low-grade infection). Thousands of healthy teeth and tonsils were removed and even large parts of the bowel. In Trenton State Hospital, New Jersey, Dr Henry Cotton championed this approach, supported by distinguished psychiatric figures right up until his death in 1933.

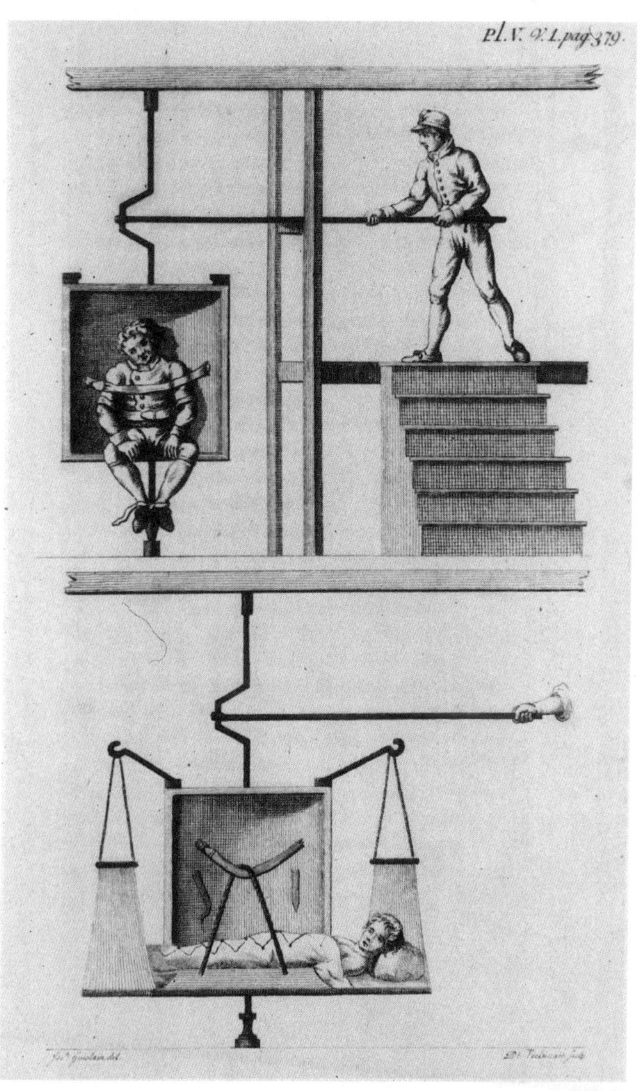

7. **Whirling chair.**

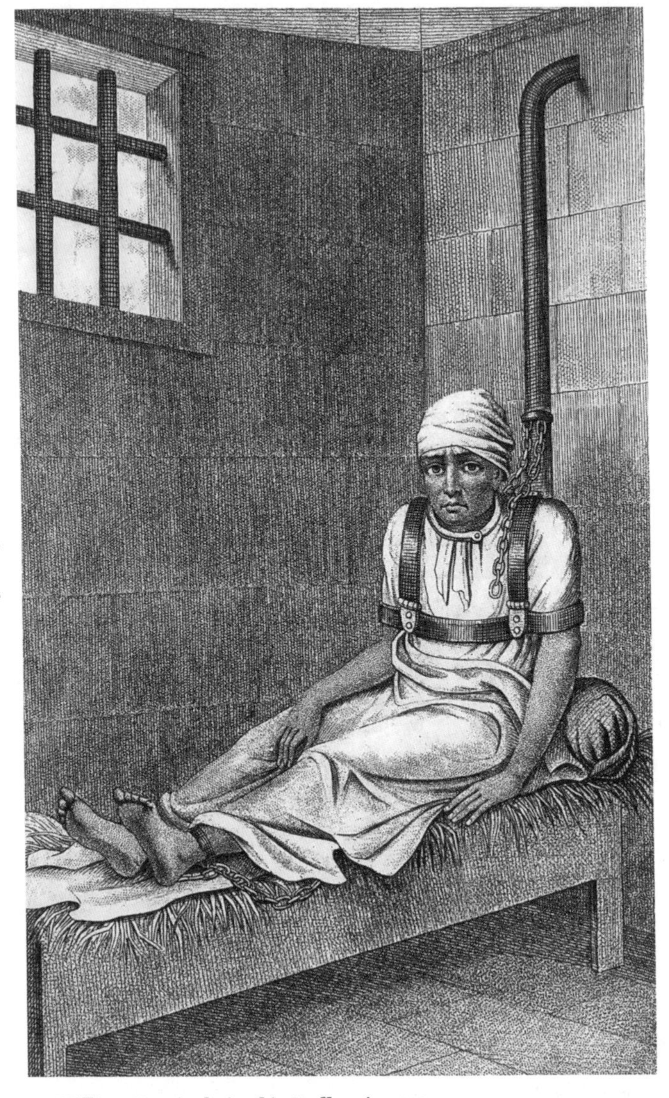

8. William Norris chained in Bedlam in 1814.

The Hawthorn effect

A special difficulty in assessing a new treatment is that the surrounding fuss and attention can itself lead to improvement. Insulin coma treatment was a case in point. Insulin had been long used in psychiatry to stimulate appetite and calm severely agitated patients (who could sometimes otherwise literally starve to death). A course of insulin comas was believed to be effective in schizophrenia and this became a common, high-prestige treatment from the 1930s through to the 1960s. It was difficult and potentially dangerous, requiring skilled and attentive nursing. It was also the first psychiatric treatment subject to a *controlled trial* to test its effect. Half the patients were put into a light sleep using tranquillizers and half into an insulin coma, without the staff knowing which was which. The results were the same for both groups, forcing the conclusion that it was the nursing attention and staff optimism that made the difference, not the insulin, and the treatment was abandoned. This effect is known as the 'Hawthorn effect' and psychiatric research always has to take account of such enthusiasm.

Enthusiasm shouldn't, however, be dismissed in psychiatry. Much of medicine may be best conducted in a dispassionate, scientific frame of mind but psychiatry requires hope and optimism from its staff. Patients are often demoralized and need help regaining hope. Hope is therapeutic in its own right as the insulin coma study indicated. Optimism has been demonstrated to affect outcome even in cancer and heart attack patients. It can, however, lead to over-enthusiasm and treatments, including effective treatments, being given well beyond their usefulness.

Electro-convulsive therapy and brain surgery

ECT was certainly overused after it was introduced in the 1930s right through to the 1960s. It continued to be used in schizophrenia and for disturbed behaviour although it had become clear that its best results were in depression. The original treatments were given without anaesthetic and it was undoubtedly sometimes misused as punishment. Sensationalist and misleading portrayals, such as the unmodified ECT given to Jack Nicholson in *One Flew Over the Cuckoo's Nest*, continue to inflame the controversy.

In many countries ECT is almost impossible to obtain in public psychiatry—in Italy, Greece, Spain, and in California in the USA. In England and several US states a ban has been proposed several times but not legislated. This is undoubtedly a result of its earlier overuse and many of its fiercest critics had received it inappropriately without benefit. However, even for those who support it, there is something off-putting. It seems such a 'crude' assault on that most delicate and mysterious of our organs, the brain. ECT is experienced as an affront to our nature as creative and sentient beings—particularly as we still do not know how it works.

Even more shocking than the overuse of ECT was the crusade of brain surgery conducted by Watts and Freeman in the early 1950s in the USA. Brain surgery in psychiatry followed the observation of a freak accident in Vermont in 1848 when a railway worker, Phineas Gage, remarkably survived an explosion firing a one-inch thick bar through his head. The only damage noted was some change in personality—he became more easy-going and unreliable, somewhat disinhibited and foul-mouthed. Surgically severing the connections to the front part of the brain (where the bar had passed through in Phineas Gage's accident) was subsequently tried on many patients as a last-ditch attempt to reduce intolerable chronic anxiety or disturbed behaviour. It is called leucotomy in Europe and lobotomy in the USA and was introduced by a Portuguese neurologist, Egas Moniz, in 1935. He received the Nobel Prize for it in 1949. Ironically, he had been wheelchair-bound from 1939 until his death in 1955 after being shot by a disgruntled schizophrenia patient.

Psychosurgery, in a much modified and reduced form, is still used to help a handful of individuals absolutely disabled with severe obsessive compulsive disorder or chronic depression. It appears to work by making the patient uninterested in their symptoms, rather than abolishing them. The patient still experiences obsessional thoughts but is able to ignore them. There are, however, still some changes in personality after the operation.

Brain surgery evokes the same disquiet as ECT. It seems altogether too invasive and brutal. The explanation of how it works is superficial and unconvincing. In the USA Freeman and Watts developed a very simple version that only required a local anaesthetic. Playing down the risks, they carried out 3,439 of these operations in large mental hospitals across the country. Between 1939 and 1951 over 50,000 such operations were performed in the USA. Modern techniques are very different (usually involving the destruction of a couple of cubic millimetres of brain tissue), highly regulated, and infrequent. Nevertheless it remains a highly charged issue where people rarely change their opinions.

Political abuse in psychiatry

Psychiatry has always had twin obligations—care for the individual patient and protection of society. This 'social control' has to be weighed carefully against individual rights, especially when using compulsion. The vastly differing psychiatric care offered to blacks in South Africa under apartheid and in the US southern states during segregation has often been characterized as political abuse. Similarly the high rate of compulsory detention of ethnic minority patients (particularly blacks of African and Caribbean origin) in England has been cited as a cultural intolerance that borders on political repression.

The use of psychiatry explicitly to repress or silence political dissidents in the former Soviet Union was, however, undoubtedly political abuse. The Soviets used a diagnosis of 'sluggish schizophrenia' to mean slowly developing withdrawal and strangeness without any positive symptoms (hallucinations, thought disorder, etc.). Sluggish schizophrenia was used to detain people with dissident political views with no clear signs of mental illness. Of course some mentally ill individuals do oppose the state, which they may believe is persecuting them. The Soviets incarcerated large numbers of clearly healthy individuals in their forensic psychiatric clinics. This scandal seriously damaged psychiatry's credibility, particularly in Central and Eastern Europe.

One positive outcome of the Soviet psychiatric abuses was the development of an international movement within psychiatry to challenge such practices. United Nations and Red Cross organizations regularly visit and monitor prisons and detention centres throughout the world and now include mental hospitals in this work. China had to submit to international scrutiny over its dealings with the Falun Gong sect. International awareness provides our strongest protection against political abuse.

Psychiatry unlimited: a diagnosis for everything

Psychiatry has moved centre stage in public health. Four mental illnesses rank in the World Health Organization's top ten global causes of lifelong disability. Depression is currently number two and predicted to be the number one by 2020. By 2014 one in every eight American adults had been treated for depression. Is this good news or bad news? Is it a long-overdue recognition reflecting reducing stigma? Or is it due to modern living and an ageing population, with greater stresses and a genuine increase in mental illnesses?

Could the rise in mental illness, indeed, be illusory? Are there other factors at play and could psychiatry be led astray if we don't keep an eye on them? Psychiatry operates now in a vastly different world. We are well equipped to deal with our 20th-century failings (professional arrogance and ignorance) but 21st-century risks may, however, stem more from psychiatrists unwittingly acting out the agendas of others (as Foucault has insisted they always have). Who else has such an agenda?

The patient

Psychiatric diagnoses arise in a dialogue between patient and doctor. The patient offers his concerns and the psychiatrist mentally tests these against the range of illnesses she knows. Both parties in this exchange can adjust the threshold for what is 'psychiatric'. How do we as individuals interpret our experiences? What do we just accept (even if unpleasant and difficult) and what do we consider to need help? We seek help from professionals much more readily now where previously we might have simply endured or turned to friends and relatives. Anxieties over child-rearing, disappointments in relationships, bereavement, and distress after trauma—all are now considered legitimate territory for professional help.

Society has rejected the stiff upper lip and embraced self-fulfilment and psychotherapy. It has become immeasurably more tolerant and decent as a result. Our emotions and inner life are taken seriously, we are encouraged to share them and 'understand our feelings'. Consequently, we seek help to understand them and relief from them.

This has led to an enormous rise in demand for counselling and psychotherapy, and also for antidepressants and other medications. Of the antidepressants taken in the UK over 90 per cent are prescribed by family doctors. Most of these are for individuals who will never see a psychiatrist and who would hardly have been considered unwell a generation ago. This is not necessarily a bad thing, as many patients benefit from these treatments, but there are risks. As treatment thresholds are lowered the risk that patients who need treatment will miss out is reduced. However, others unlikely to benefit will get unnecessary treatments. Relying on medicines may also distract us from exploring alternative coping skills. Persisting with an unhappy marriage and hoping that pills will make it better is not a sensible long-term plan. Also, as social expectations change imperceptibly personal resilience may be eroded.

Treatments we seek from psychiatrists may even make us worse. Excessive prescription of valium and other sedatives led to an epidemic of dependence which proved enormously difficult to reverse. Routine counselling after disasters has been shown to slow down recovery. Perhaps some experiences are best simply put behind one. In natural disasters, counselling may divert energy and attention away from more beneficial social cohesion and family support.

'Big Pharma'

There is a growing unease about the relationship of the medical profession with the companies which research, manufacture, and sell the drugs we use. The cost of developing a prescription drug in the USA is estimated at $2,500,000,000 in 2015. So the pharmaceutical industry is increasingly concentrated in a small group of immensely powerful multinational businesses. The statistics are staggering. It takes on average up to ten years from patenting a drug, via tests and trials, to first prescriptions. Only 1 per cent of new molecules make it from test tube to prescription.

Not surprising then that the marketing of these drugs is ruthless. The financial relationships between doctors and these companies are murky. Pharmaceutical companies have routinely offered luxurious hospitality and travel to doctors as barely concealed inducement for prescribing. Europe has recently cracked down on this, but the practice is still widespread globally. Until recently psychiatry was relatively immune from this as our drugs cost so little.

However, the new generation antipsychotics and antidepressants are vastly more expensive. The newer 'atypical' antipsychotics cost several thousand dollars a year per patient in the USA compared to a couple of hundred or less for the older drugs; newer antidepressants also cost several hundred dollars a year as opposed to pennies for the older tricyclic antidepressants. The patent on a new drug is strictly time limited and the companies have to recoup all their development costs usually within 10–15 years from launch. With the financial muscle of the pharmaceutical companies invested in drugs, it is hardly surprising that social and psychological treatments without such financial backing struggle.

'Big Pharma' has been accused of stretching the boundaries of what are treatable psychiatric disorders to increase the sales of its drugs. It has been accused of creating 'illnesses for drugs' rather than developing 'drugs for illnesses'. The enormous success of Prozac has led to an expansion of the concept of clinical depression with milder and milder cases treated. Prozac's iconic status undoubtedly helped reduce the stigma of depression but also made it something of a 'lifestyle' drug. Most university students will know class-mates on antidepressants—inconceivable only a generation ago. Diagnostic patterns have changed in response to the marketing of these drugs. There is a striking increase in the diagnosis of disorders such as PTSD (post-traumatic stress disorder) and social phobia (a disorder which some would consider just extreme shyness) once drugs are licensed to treat them.

Even more worrying is the massive growth in psychiatric prescribing for children. Once a rarity, child psychiatrists now regularly prescribe psychotropic drugs. The most dramatic increase has been in the diagnosis and treatment of ADHD (attention deficit hyperactivity disorder): in the USA 11 per cent of schoolchildren (3 per cent in the UK) and 4 per cent of adults are diagnosed with ADHD, with over half on stimulant drugs.

The prescribing of Ritalin (methylphenidate) increased sixfold in the 1990s in the USA and accounts for 85 per cent of world prescriptions, but Europe is rapidly catching up, doubling in the last decade in the UK with one million prescriptions in 2016. Irrespective of the controversy about the legitimacy of the diagnosis, there can be little doubt that psychiatric practice is being fuelled at least partly by commercial agendas.

Before leaving the pharmaceutical industry we need to acknowledge its very positive contribution to human health and welfare. The drugs *do* work. It would be naive to ignore the financial imperatives that flow from such staggering R&D costs and to profess surprise at the marketing practices. The dramatic increase in both its scale and power, however, raise ethical problems which are not restricted to psychiatry. They include the exploitation of poorer countries for research where ethical standards may be less strict and where the patients in these trials may never have the resources to benefit from the drugs developed. The temptation to create spurious health needs to sell products is particularly potent in the psychological sphere as almost everyone would like to 'feel a bit better'. Honest debate and tighter guidelines are urgently needed.

Reliability versus validity

Diagnosis in psychiatry has moved towards a criterion-based system (see the diagnostic criteria for depression in Chapter 1). Traditionally diagnosis was based on pattern recognition informed by extensive familiarity with normal and abnormal behaviours. This is being replaced by a careful listing of features of the disorder that are present. The change was a response to unacceptable variations in diagnostic practice. The new diagnostic system (pioneered in the 1980 Diagnostic and Statistical Manual—DSM III, now in the 2013 DSM5) aimed to remove reliance on psychiatric theories which had previously caused regular disagreements. Whether one really can have an entirely 'atheoretical' diagnostic system is, of course, questionable.

The new system emphasizes *reliability* more than *validity*. Reliability ensures that different psychiatrists faced with the same symptoms will always come to the same diagnosis whereas validity ensures that patients with the same diagnosis would have similar outcomes and responses to treatment. The goal would be, of course, maximum reliability and maximum validity. Unfortunately, good reliability does not necessarily guarantee validity. The fact that we all agree on certain defining characteristics doesn't mean it really is 'something'. An extreme example is 17th-century witch-finders. They were very reliable—they consistently agreed on all the tell-tale signs of a witch before they burnt her. Despite their reliability we would dispute their validity in identifying a witch.

Reliability can mistakenly imply validity so that a condition gets accorded the status of a diagnosis essentially because psychiatrists can agree on how to define and recognize it. We have already encountered a couple of these controversial diagnoses—social phobia and ADHD—but there are several more which really stretch credibility. Nicotine and caffeine 'use disorders' are now both official psychiatric diagnoses in DSM5, but few of us would consider these mental illnesses. Similarly, there is a range of behavioural patterns which have acquired the highly questionable status of a diagnosis (and therefore may receive 'treatment'—an important commercial consideration in some health care systems). An example is DSM5's 'oppositional defiant disorder', diagnosed by an angry or irritable mood with persistent defiance and episodes of arguing with authority figures, refusing to comply with requests, losing their temper, or blaming others, which is suspiciously close to the description of a difficult teenager.

Psychiatric gullibility

Psychiatrists on the whole are trusting souls. We tend to take our patients' stories at face value. This was vividly demonstrated in the notorious 'Being Sane in Insane Places' study. In 1973 eight volunteers attended emergency rooms in America complaining of a voice in their head which simply said 'empty', 'hollow', or 'thud'. All eight were admitted to psychiatric units where they then behaved absolutely normally. Amazingly they remained in hospital for an average of just under three weeks and, worse still, most still had a diagnosis on discharge of 'schizophrenia in remission'. Not surprising then that there was such a demand for better diagnosis in the 1980 DSM III.

So there are several forces to drive diagnostic expansion acting on psychiatry beyond the natural curiosity of researchers. Whether this is desirable should not be left to the profession alone to decide. It requires debate within the broader society (i.e. you).

Personality problems and addictions

Psychiatrists have always dealt with the consequences of drug and alcohol addictions. They have also always encountered personalities which are strikingly unusual and can cause endless problems. The level of distress and disruption associated with such personalities is beyond dispute, and these individuals often concentrate in mental health services. There is, however, a legitimate dispute about whether they should be considered psychiatric disorders in themselves and whether psychiatrists should be responsible for treating them. This is not a trivial matter as they may sometimes be treated against their wishes.

Coercion in psychiatry

Compulsory treatment (treatment imposed against explicit refusal by the patient) is permitted within psychiatry in every society. This includes Western societies whose fundamental principles include respect for individual liberty before the law. The handling of mental illness is a very striking exception. Mental illnesses may involve a clear 'break' with normal functioning that estranges the patient from their usual self. This is unlike learning disability where the individual may have never developed the capacity to make informed and competent decisions. The striking characteristic of mental illnesses is a *change*. Most societies have sanctioned a paternalistic provision for coercive treatment from a humane desire to protect an individual who is clearly 'not themselves'. This is supported by the observation that most patients recover and many express the same concerns as the rest of us about their behaviour when they were unwell. Many even express gratitude that they were compulsorily treated.

Lawyers find these areas difficult. The standard assessment of 'capacity' to make treatment decisions is the ability to *understand* the information, the ability to *trust* the individual giving the information, and the ability to *retain* and make a decision based on that information. This scheme works well for children, the learning disabled, and those with dementia. However, it doesn't work well where the problem is one of judgement and mood rather than intellectual ability or logical reasoning. Imposing treatment against a patient's will rests ultimately on the psychiatrist's conclusion that the patient is suffering from a mental illness such that their current decisions are not those they would usually make. Note that this involves the psychiatrist making a judgement on what he believes that the patient would *usually do* or want when well. Compulsion is also sometimes used as a brief safety measure with people not clearly mentally ill but who are 'temporarily unbalanced'—a terrified individual in a strange place or a young person attempting to kill or harm themselves in despair after a relationship break-up.

Severe personality disorders

Psychiatry's attitude to psychopathic and antisocial personality disorder (usually in men), and borderline personality disorder (usually in women), is also problematic. Psychopaths are cold, callous individuals who lack empathy for others and consequently can commit awful crimes. They give no thought to the consequences for others and show no remorse afterwards. They are often recognizable early on (death of pets, arson, etc.). Being self-centred and not caring about others' feelings, they can be extremely successful; it is jokingly proposed that mild psychopathy is essential for being a successful politician. Psychopaths are often lumped together with explosive and violent individuals as antisocial personality disorder. This group poses a massive problem for prisons and the criminal justice system.

In some countries psychiatrists detain these individuals under the same conditions as the mentally ill and this has been criticized as an abuse of power. To justify coercion the condition is usually considered time-limited and there is some confidence that the treatment will speed recovery. Neither of these conditions are met for severe personality disorders. Their behaviour reflects their personality—their real identity, nothing aberrant or temporary. And, unfortunately, to date there is no convincing evidence that forced treatments will significantly change that. Such people pose profound challenges for society and psychiatrists debate endlessly whether compulsory (or indeed any) treatment is indicated.

In the first edition of this book I wrote that 'the Western world has experienced an upsurge in chaotic self-damaging behaviour in young women'. This is now a global phenomenon—albeit not quite so common everywhere. Overdosing and cutting have become extremely common among women in mental hospitals and prisons. Such patients seem out of control, are clearly distressed, and damage themselves in what often seems like a mixture of anger and a desperate plea for help. Psychiatrists feel responsible but impotent and often try to 'contain' the situation by keeping the patient compulsorily on a ward offering supervision and support. Unfortunately, things often go from bad to worse—the patient self-harms more and the psychiatrist increases the restrictions to control the situation. Alongside calls for improved youth mental health services to help these women, some pressure groups argue that what these women do to their bodies is their own affair and psychiatry is overstepping the mark in treating them against their will. They point to the cultural precedents for self-mutilation such as religious and ritual scarring and underline how medicine, and psychiatry in particular, has consistently denied women's self-determination over their own bodies.

Drug and alcohol abuse

A similar set of arguments holds for drug and alcohol abuse. Both can be associated with mental illness and both can also cause mental illnesses. Fine for psychiatry to be involved then. But are drug or alcohol abuse mental illnesses in themselves? The rebranding of addictions as illnesses was a humanitarian impulse in the 1930s. Alcoholics Anonymous, founded in 1939, provides help to support addicted individuals and promote sobriety. Alcoholics Anonymous (AA) and Narcotics Anonymous (NA) are the world's largest self-help groups and consider addiction a lifelong, incurable illness, although they rely on personal and spiritual support rather than medical treatment.

AA and NA view the addict as fundamentally different from other individuals, never able to use drugs or alcohol safely. Within psychiatry, however, there are divided views. For some addiction is an illness to be treated like any other, while others view drug and alcohol abuse as dangerous habits that can lead to mental illnesses but are not themselves helpfully understood as illnesses. They are ultimately the individual's own responsibility, as they can exert direct influence on their condition in a way that is not possible for someone with depression or schizophrenia. Medicalization of substance abuse is considered a distraction from effective public health measures, such as raising the price and restricting access, which have been repeatedly shown to successfully reduce drinking and drink-related illness and death.

Offering help such as prescribing medicines to cope with withdrawal and support to build up a sober lifestyle are generally uncontroversial, unlike the use of compulsion. In much of Scandinavia, Eastern Europe, and Russia there has been extensive use of specialized mental hospitals for longer-term detention of alcoholics and drug addicts. Can this be justified? The consequences of heavy drinking or drug abuse can undoubtedly be disastrous, even fatal. But many of us make foolish decisions and suffer the consequences—smoking is more dangerous to health than drinking, but we don't compulsorily treat smokers. The confused thinking and poor judgement when intoxicated is also a questionable justification for psychiatric intervention as some of the attraction of intoxication is precisely to alter judgements by blurring an unwelcome reality.

Increasing sophistication in genetics and epidemiology has helped identify those who are at greater risk of alcoholism and drug abuse. There are well-recognized ethnic variations in the ability to tolerate and metabolize alcohol. These findings strengthen the contention that these are not lifestyle choices but disorders. The issue remains open and psychiatry's role in drug and alcohol abuse will remain controversial.

The insanity defence

Criticisms of coercion in psychiatry concern unfairly depriving individuals of their rights. Mental health legislation, however, was also introduced to protect patients from severe punishment for crimes committed while unwell. Society has always felt uncomfortable about such punishments. The crime of infanticide was separated from murder because 19th-century juries simply refused to send to the hangman mothers who killed their babies while suffering post-partum psychoses.

The importance of establishing criminal intent ('mens rea' or 'guilty mind') has guaranteed a long and tortured relationship between psychiatrists and the courts. Agreeing whether or not someone was insane at the time of the crime (i.e. unable to judge the significance of their acts and realize that they were wrong) has in principle been fairly straightforward. However, it is often far from easy in the individual case. Floridly ill patients, unable to understand court proceedings, may be judged unfit to plead and admitted directly to hospital for treatment. Most countries will accept the decision of unfit to plead on the basis of a psychiatric assessment or will return a not-guilty verdict on the grounds of insanity.

The real problems in court concern diminished responsibility on the grounds of mental illness. This is particularly so where the criminal behaviour itself may be the first or the clearest manifestation of the disorder. It is less a problem with a grossly disturbed individual whose crime is just one among many signs of the illness. An easy example would be a manic patient in court for reckless driving, but who is rude to the magistrate, is dressed bizarrely, not sleeping, and has been spending all his money. Advancing personality disorders as a defence is invariably problematic. Proposing that because a psychopath does not notice or care about the distress caused he should not be held criminally responsible and punished strikes at the concept of free will and personal responsibility, which is the very foundation of criminal justice thinking. Most criminals have had dreadful childhoods. Many have been abused. Few have skilled jobs or stable families to fall back upon. So it is not surprising that we may temper justice with mercy. But there is a circularity in citing the very qualities that give rise to the crime as a justification for a reduced punishment. This ethical dilemma is particularly sharp in individuals with Asperger's syndrome (a mild form of autism) who cannot see the world from another's perspective and cannot interpret others' motives even though they may desperately want to.

In practice the more serious the crime and the greater the risk, the easier the decision. Where the alternative to a guilty verdict and prison is hospital care (and sometimes prolonged secure hospital care) courts and juries feel more comfortable to make the allowance. In lesser cases, where punishment is not so severe, and might just deter repeat offending, a psychiatric defence may do the individual no favour in the long term. Thomas Szasz (Chapter 5) insisted that the psychiatric defence is a denial of the fundamental rights and obligations of the individual. A psychiatric defence is generally accepted for individuals where the disorder is plainly there for all to see.

Sometimes the only evidence of a disorder is the crime. In several high-profile cases of murder the perpetrator has denied any memory, claiming it occurred during an 'automatism' (a dream-like or dissociated state). In even more extreme cases 'multiple personalities' have been proposed where a single individual has several fully developed identities, each completely independent of each other. This concept, a Dr Jekyll and Mr Hyde, appeals strongly to popular imagination.

The suggested mechanism is that some mental processes are so successfully repressed that they are only accessible through deep psychotherapy or 'triggered' in highly specific situations. This is of enormous psychiatric/legal significance in cases of alleged childhood sexual abuse. To what extent children are exposed to sexual abuse by family members has long been controversial in psychiatry. The pendulum has swung back and forth between considering it a common trauma that causes neuroses to the alternative belief that it is rare and most reports are 'false memories'. Currently the presumption is strongly in favour of believing the adult who complains of earlier sexual abuse. This has resulted in high-profile cases splitting families when 'recovered memories' have been unearthed. Psychiatrists appear on both sides of the case, stressing either the damaging impact of abuse, repressed over many years, or, conversely, the patient's suggestibility in over-enthusiastic therapy.

Psychiatry: a controversial practice

The examples given here are just some of the reasons psychiatric practice will always be risky and controversial. Many psychiatrists argue for a safer, more limited, approach restricted to well-established mental illnesses. 'We should stick to treating diagnosed illnesses, schizophrenia, anorexia nervosa, depression and recognize there are many causes of human distress besides mental illness. Leave social policy and ethics to politicians and philosophers.' This is an attractive argument. The history of psychiatry is full of examples of overstepping the mark. But as we have seen in this chapter it is not simply up to psychiatrists—there are other stakeholders and powerful forces at play. We confront knotty ethical dilemmas with significant potential benefits in the balance.

Scientific developments are expanding what we can do; families and patients have steadily rising expectations from us; governments and the pharmaceutical industry challenge us with new demands, inducements, and opportunities. The only way to avoid controversy and the possibility of mistakes would be to turn our backs on progress and innovation. But that would mean abandoning psychiatry's promise and its obligations. Psychiatry straddles hard science and the field of human behaviour and ambitions, so it is simply impossible to be uncontroversial. It comes with the territory and, as we explore in Chapter 7, these challenges may be getting greater.

Chapter 7
Into the 21st century

New technologies and old dilemmas

It is risky to make predictions. How would Albert Einstein's teacher look back on his 1895 report: 'It doesn't matter what he does, he'll never amount to anything'? Or the editor of *Popular Mechanics* in 1949: 'Computers in future may weigh no more than 1.5 tons.' We know how Decca Records regretted their judgement on the Beatles in 1962: 'We don't like their sound, and guitar music is on the way out.'

Psychiatry in the first quarter of the 21st century is very different from that of just a few decades ago. Nobody ever imagined that we would be able to record brain activity in real time and in detail. Now we are able to watch as different areas of this notoriously 'silent' organ light up demonstrating its activity in such varied functions as initiating movement or registering sights and sounds—even hallucinatory perceptions! Enormous and accelerating advances in genetics and neuroscience dazzle us with insights into the bases of mental processes and the mechanisms underlying our vulnerabilities. Changes in computer technology and the advent of the digital age affect how we relate to each other, and consequently our experience of mental illness and how we can try to help.

Optimists believe that these advances may soon eradicate mental illnesses altogether or, at the very least, make our treatments so rational and uncontroversial that we will simply blend into general medicine. Others point to the paradox of increasing compulsion and rising suicide rates despite better treatments. New ethical challenges arise from improved genetic prediction and the marginalization of the disabled by a high-tech and increasingly mobile society. Ironically, the very rapidity of scientific advances within neuroscience has stimulated a resurgence of interest in social psychiatry and psychological understanding.

As the quotes at the start of this chapter confirm, it is notoriously difficult to pick a winner, but there are some likely front-runners. A striking change since the first edition of this book is an increased focus on how our body, and not just the brain, influences our mental health. Rapidly advancing computer technology is also beginning to provide new treatment possibilities, not just support and simplify the old ones.

Neuroscience

Neurosciences have become 'the hot topic' in medical research. The development of sophisticated imaging has supercharged the area. Primitive methods of visualizing the brain such as X-rays and air encephalography (injecting air into the fluid filled spaces in the brain to outline deep structures) could identify gross distortions such as tumours and strokes. They could also confirm extensive shrinkage of the brain in dementia, but on the whole they were far too crude to be of much value in psychiatry. CAT scanning (Computer Assisted Tomography) provides multiple X-ray 'slices' of the brain so that a detailed 3-D picture can be created. MRI (Magnetic Resonance Imaging) also produces such detailed 3-D pictures and, lacking the risks of repeated X-rays, can be used to measure changes over time.

Even the most detailed understanding of brain structure, however, remains of limited value in psychiatry. Our major disorders (schizophrenia, depression, etc.) used to be referred to as 'functional' disorders to stress the absence of any detectable anatomical abnormality. fMRI (Functional MRI) introduced in the late 1990s records the *activity* of brain areas. fMRI produces its images by detecting increased blood flow, oxygen uptake, and glucose metabolism with remarkable precision (the brain is a hungry organ utilizing 20 per cent of our daily calories). fMRI has already led to some striking discoveries such as demonstrating that hallucinatory experiences involve the same brain activity as real perceptions. It has also aided localization of brain areas with increased or reduced activity in some disorders. This has prompted work on implanting electric wires to stimulate activity in depression and Parkinson's disease. fMRI has also confirmed the enormous complexity and interconnectedness of brain activity and is regularly used in psychological experiments to map the regions involved in complicated responses.

These developments hold great promise but are still a long way from the 'Cyborg' fantasy of inserting small computer chips to control behaviour. Indeed, there is a noticeable reluctance among scientists to apply invasive techniques such as surgery and cell transplantation in mental illnesses as they are used in neurological disorders. Because they pose such fundamental challenges to our selfhood and personal identity they generate caution and require very careful ethical consideration.

Genetics

Psychiatrists have always taken genetics seriously. However, psychiatric disorders do not follow the simple Mendelian patterns of dominant and recessive inheritance we learnt about in school (Huntington's disease is the striking exception). The failure to follow these simple laws in diseases such as schizophrenia and manic depression, despite overwhelming evidence of hereditability, has been the source of the endless nature–nurture disputes. Modern genetics, starting with Watson and Crick's clarification of the double helix structure of DNA in 1953, has become vastly more sophisticated. We can now map the location of individual genes on our chromosomes. The Human Genome Project started in 1990 and had mapped the entire human genetic sequence by 2003. Automation of the process now means that any of us can sequence our genes and obtain disease risks within a few weeks for only a few pounds.

Modern psychiatric genetics has abandoned the search for 'the schizophrenia gene'. We know there isn't one, but probably around two hundred genes that contribute to the risk for the disease. Neuregulin 1 (a gene identified in schizophrenia families in Iceland and the west of Scotland) is probably a *necessary* condition for developing the disease but not a *sufficient* one (about 30 per cent of us carry it). Understanding these complicated genetics involves the new science of epigenetics, which studies the impact of other genes and environmental triggers to activate specific genes. Within psychiatry this improved sophistication of genetic mapping interacts with social psychiatry. For example, genes known to raise the risk of depression have been shown in long-term follow-up studies to only have an effect if the person was also exposed to marked adversity in childhood. Without that stress the gene seems to remain inactive.

Early identification

Improved understanding of genetic risk factors is changing the already controversial practice of early identification. In families with a schizophrenic member, researchers in Australia have examined siblings for signs of vulnerability long before any clear symptoms arise. Such 'ultra high risk' individuals are usually a bit withdrawn and 'odd' and may report unusual, but not frankly psychotic, experiences. Trials of starting treatment with antipsychotic medication and psychological support before the illness manifests itself claim to have prevented a substantial number of 'transitions' (i.e. developing into the full disorder). It does not take much imagination to realize the emotional minefield this opens up for young people at such a sensitive period. Not surprisingly, this approach has not become routine, but with the increased precision of modern genetics and epigenetics it can surely only be a matter of time—and not just for schizophrenia.

Treating people who have never had any symptoms may become an even knottier problem as drug development becomes more sophisticated. Even with the advent of Prozac a couple of decades ago the question of 'lifestyle' drugs arose when some patients described being on it as 'better than well'. Just as the world of sport is struggling to find a position on performance enhancing drugs, the same issues are arising with 'smart drugs' that enhance intellectual performance. Some of the drugs used for ADHD improve thinking even if you don't have a psychiatric problem, and their use is widespread among students. Is this fair or is it cheating? More importantly, is it a sensible way to conduct our lives? Presumably the same will happen as drugs to slow down dementia improve and people want them as a form of insurance.

Whole body psychiatry

There is an upsurge in research beyond neuroscience exploring the impact of our physical health on mental well-being. This goes beyond recognizing the value of exercise in delaying dementia and improving mood, or identifying physical processes in the brain. Probably the most surprising is work on the bacteria in our gut (referred to as either microbiota or the microbiome). These bacteria are so numerous that in each individual they weigh more than our brain and produce a number of known psychoactive substances. Their direct impact on mental states has been repeatedly shown in experimental animals. Anxiety and depressive states in some strains of mice can be completely reversed by substituting different microbes in their gut. In humans there are some suggestions that different bacteria profiles are also associated with depression and anxiety.

The link between psychological functioning and the immune system has long been a focus of interest as our awareness of the sensitivity of both to stress has grown. As this book goes to press there is a study of treating acutely ill schizophrenia patients with monthly infusions of a chemotherapy drug which acts on the immune system and is hoped to modify mental processes. This is all very exciting stuff. However, we should not forget that promises of such radical treatments and dramatic potential breakthroughs have been present throughout psychiatry's history.

Computers and psychiatry

Computers have changed just about everything in our lives and that includes psychiatry. Over the last twenty years they have supported existing treatments and practices, making them more efficient and readily available. There are dozens of examples. We have digitalized mental state monitoring—depressed patients can record their mood on their smart phone daily and then examine the resultant coloured patterns to spot early warnings of breakdowns. An antipsychotic pill is already available that broadcasts to a smartphone to confirm when it is taken! Web and app-based CBT programmes are popular for a number of conditions from anxiety to depression and eating disorders. Younger patients, having grown up with computers, obviously take better to these approaches. iPads are being used to give real-time feedback in consultations of the match between the patient's assessment of their needs and the therapist's. All of these, and more, are essentially using computing to support and improve established practices. However, we are now moving into an era when computers will be delivering innovations that are unique to them and which, even with unlimited time and effort, we could never match.

Artificial intelligence (AI)

Medicine, like the rest of society, is bracing itself for the impact of artificial intelligence. With big data and powerful computers human clinical judgement can now often be surpassed with more accurate predictions and, disconcertingly, more personalized predictions and treatment regimes. This should not really surprise us. AI utilizes the same process as traditional medical education—adding layer of experience upon layer of experience to improve pattern recognition and discrimination, and then fitting that to the patient in front of you. The only difference is that the computer can learn from the experience of hundreds of doctors with thousands of patients. AI is radically different from earlier forms of computer-assisted learning as the computer can review and rewrite its algorithms itself as it acquires more 'knowledge'. Some of our preconceptions with which we primed the programme are abandoned and replaced with new ones that we may be utterly unaware of. As with driverless cars we have to relinquish our preconceptions that machines can only deal with the commonplace and predictable. Chess-playing computers have defeated even the most creative grandmasters. The computer may become even better than us at applying in-depth experience to novel and unusual, highly personal, situations.

Virtual reality

The ability of computers to control what we experience in simulated situations is already in use in psychiatry. Virtual reality (VR) programmes can provide an artificial but convincingly real environment that can be repeated exactly from patient to patient allowing a detailed understanding of how reality is interpreted. Figure 9 shows a VR scenario in a tube train where the patient can look around the carriage and observe a number of people moving and interacting and then be questioned about the experience. This programme quickly identifies our different ways of interpreting the world around us. Paranoid individuals read sinister motives

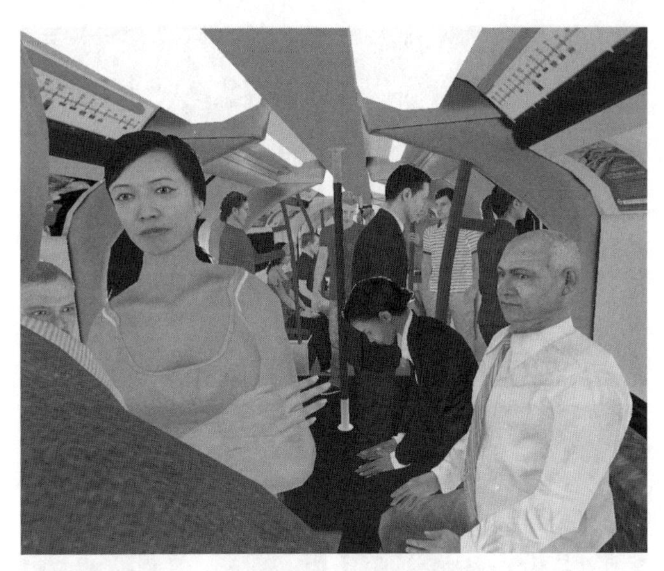

9. Virtual reality interior of London Underground train carriage. Patients are asked to describe what they see in the VR experience of a tube carriage and explain the behaviour of those around them.

into some of the neutral figures ('Why is he looking round at me like that? Why did he look away suddenly?'). Treatments are already in development based on activities conducted within VR.

One such development is 'Avatar' treatment for schizophrenia patients tormented by hallucinations (Figure 10). The patient gives a detailed description of the appearance, voice, and behaviour of the person they think is responsible for the voices in their head. An 'identikit' version is made of the face and the sound of the voice (accent, intonation). Then using sophisticated software the voice and facial expressions of a therapist are transformed to those of this persecuting figure in real time. Patients are encouraged to get into dialogue with the voices which they experience as from the avatar on the screen but whose words are in reality spoken (and then transformed) by the therapist. They can then challenge the content

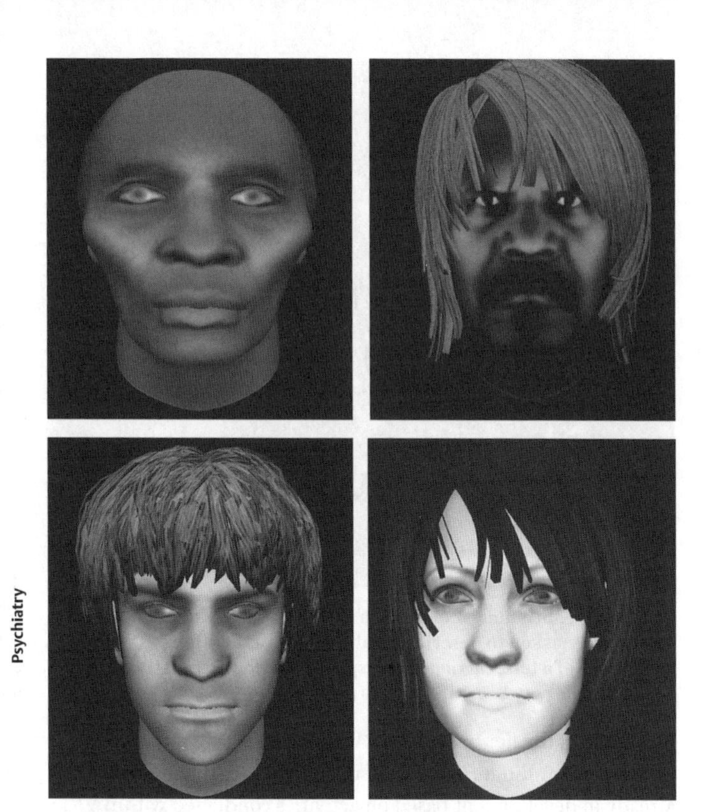

10. Avatar faces used in treatment of hallucinations.

of the hallucinations and develop some control and distance. Early results show that the frequency, intensity, and fearfulness of these voices can be reduced.

Social, psychological, and biological balance

A paradox with our increasingly technological and scientific advances is that the core dilemmas of psychiatry appear not to be diminishing. If anything they are intensifying. Compulsion is increasing worldwide and services find themselves (despite expanding resources and staffing) even more stretched to meet demand. Partly this is because of a widening of psychiatry's diagnostic reach, but it is not just that.

Psychiatry is being forced to change in response to broader changes in society. We live much less predictable lives, often in fragmented communities and families. Little can be taken for granted—even gender is becoming fluid. Most modern societies consist of individuals with widely different cultures, expectations, and often origins including the challenge of millions of displaced people. Just as care in the community has become a reality the traditional carers in that community (mothers and wives) have opted for a life in the workplace. With increased longevity families find themselves caring for elderly frail parents at the same time they support children and grandchildren.

Changes in psychiatry are driven as much, if not more, by changes in society rather than technological advances. Social psychiatry (the exploration of how the wider social network impacts patients and how the environment can be changed to promote recovery and resilience) is making something of a come-back. Prominent in the 1950s and 1960s it had been overshadowed by biomedical psychiatry in recent decades.

This risk that psychiatry may invade all aspects of our life and 'medicalize' the human condition is increased by the emphasis on the simpler, more reliable but democratically negotiated, approach to diagnosis discussed in Chapter 6. The size of the psychiatric population used to be restricted by psychiatrists only giving a diagnosis when the patient's experience and behaviour was felt to be fundamentally 'different'. If a diagnosis follows automatically from a series of complaints (without being filtered through such a judgement), then there is little restriction on expansion. We increasingly encourage self-disclosure and attention to our feelings, hence perhaps the rapidly rising number of people who consider themselves depressed or anxious. Most of us welcome this more accepting, open approach to human experience. Equally, most of us support a more balanced relationship embodied in a psychiatric consultation which takes the patient's symptoms more seriously than the psychiatrist's preoccupations. But are we happy with the consequences as ever-widening segments of our lives become labelled as psychiatric disorder?

Old dilemmas in new forms

Despite all our progress we have entered the 21st century with remarkably similar dilemmas to those on entering the 20th. Compulsion in psychiatry has not gone away—rather increased somewhat. Similarly, the fear that psychiatry may trivialize individual differences and treat people as objects remains just as strong. This conflict may now be played out between 'evidence based medicine' versus 'post-modern individualism', where once it was the crushing uniformity of large asylums versus the dignity of the patient. Society and psychiatry will always have (and probably always *should* have) an uneasy relationship balancing duty to the patients and duty to society. The very durability of these debates reveals them as not simply technical problems. They show how psychiatry is so intimately bound up with what it is to be truly human. They reflect the tensions and paradoxes that are inherent to psychiatry as a discipline and with which we started this book.

Will psychiatry survive the 21st century?

The imminent demise of psychiatry has been predicted for most of its history. Optimists anticipate dramatic breakthroughs that will tame mental illnesses in the way that antibiotics defeated tuberculosis or vaccination eradicated smallpox. The mental hygiene movement also hoped that rational child care, reduced alcohol consumption, and improved social conditions would make the analyst and psychotherapist redundant. It hasn't happened. The very success of modern medicine has brought with it the challenges of an ageing population with increasing depression and the ticking time-bomb of Alzheimer's disease. Greater openness and respect for individual feelings have resulted in an enormous increase in the demand for counselling and psychotherapy. The numbers of psychiatrists and mental health professionals has risen inexorably across the world. On this simple head-count of staff and the mounting demand for its service, yes, it should continue to flourish.

But will it survive as it is now? Certainly things are changing. Might the psychological and psychotherapeutic treatments separate from the more traditionally medical treatment of the psychoses? In many parts of the world psychiatry has only recently gained its independence from neurology, but we now hear strong calls for reuniting them as a logical development of a more powerful medical psychiatry for the future. Many psychiatrists already call themselves 'neuropsychiatrists' and some suggest replacing the title altogether with 'clinical neuroscientists'. In several health care systems psychiatrists deal almost exclusively with diagnosis and inpatient care, based on a biomedical model. Long-term outpatient care of disabled patients is meanwhile managed by social workers and psychologists/psychotherapists using a more interpersonal approach. These pressures are not new, but with many highly trained clinical psychologists, nurses, and social workers available the power structures are shifting and radically different practices evolving.

There is a logic to such developments. Increased knowledge drives specialization, so some fragmentation of psychiatry is inevitable. Despite this, psychiatry flourishes. Departments of psychiatry are still seen as a measure of progress. When people can choose they still seem to prefer that mixture of medical expertise (or is it authority?) combined with psychological and emotional sensitivity traditional to psychiatry. Psychiatry's medical pedigree gives reassurance, yet few of us believe that it is really *just* a branch of medicine.

The mind is not the same as the brain. The defining characteristic of mental illnesses (and consequently psychiatry) remains their impact on our sense of who we are and on our closest relationships. Working with these is the hallmark of psychiatry, however it is configured, and there is no evidence of society losing interest in it. There probably will be a *Very Short Introduction to Psychiatry* in fifty years' time.

Further reading

This VSI has been a whirlwind tour round psychiatry. It *does not* aim to give a technical or professional understanding of the subject, nor to give advice about what to do for a psychiatric problem you think you or someone close to you may have. Hopefully, you will feel able to approach a professional and will realize that there is a tolerant and welcoming reception for you if you do. Here are a few suggestions for those who want to read more.

Chapter 1: What is psychiatry?

Geddes, J., Price, J., and McKnight, R., *Psychiatry* (OUP, 2012)

There are several textbooks of psychiatry, but even the best of them is written to accompany practical training and my inclination would not be to recommend one. However, if you really do want to look up a specific illness or problem, then I would currently recommend a textbook rather than the web, which can be very confusing.

Burns, Tom, *Our Necessary Shadow: The Nature and Meaning of Psychiatry* (Penguin, 2014). Covers the same ground as this book but in much greater detail.

Chapters 2: Asylums and the origins of psychiatry and 3: The move into the community

Porter, Roy, *Madness: A Brief History* (OUP, 2002)
Shorter, Edward, *A History of Psychiatry* (Wiley, 1997)
Jones, Kathleen, *Asylums and After* (Athlone Press, 1993)

Almost anything by the late Roy Porter is worth reading on the history of asylums (which he called 'museums of madness'). Shorter is even more critical of the profession. Kathleen Jones's book is the classic and more balanced but no longer in print, though obtainable through libraries. All are entertaining, but each has a definite perspective.

Chapter 4: Psychoanalysis and psychotherapy

Burns, Tom and Burns-Lundgren, Eva, *Psychotherapy: A Very Short Introduction* (OUP, 2015)

Companion volume to this one, but focusing on the varieties of psychotherapy and counselling.

Storr, Anthony, *Freud: A Very Short Introduction* (OUP, 2001)
Stevens, Anthony, *Jung: A Very Short Introduction* (OUP, 2001)

These are two short, jargon-free introductions to the two most dominant figures in the psychoanalytical movement.

Chapter 5: Psychiatry under attack—inside and out

Laing, R. D., *The Divided Self* (Penguin Books, 1960)
Foucault, Michel, *Madness and Civilization* (Tavistock Publications, 1961)
Bentall, Richard, *Madness Explained: Psychosis and Human Nature* (Penguin Books, 2003)

The Divided Self is the iconic anti-psychiatry text of the 1960s. Foucault is much harder to read. Bentall brings the debate up to the minute with a more scientific, less philosophical, approach, but which is still very challenging. All these books are still in print.

Chapter 6: Open to abuse

Porter's and Shorter's books have lots to say about these issues too. Erving Goffman, *Asylums* (Anchor, 1961), is rather long but very insightful about a range of human activities and led the charge against the asylums by exposing malpractice.

Index

Page numbers in italics refer to illustrations.

C

D

R

S